Why we

Home workouts

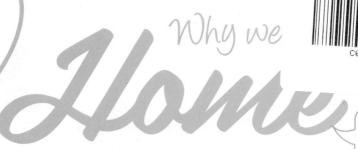

C000231450

You don't have to
wait for a shower

It's free

There's no commute

3

You don't have to worry about what you
look like – no one's watching you

**You can wear
what you like**

**There's no
forgetting
your
underwear**

There's no need
for gym small talk

**You don't have
to share a
changing room**

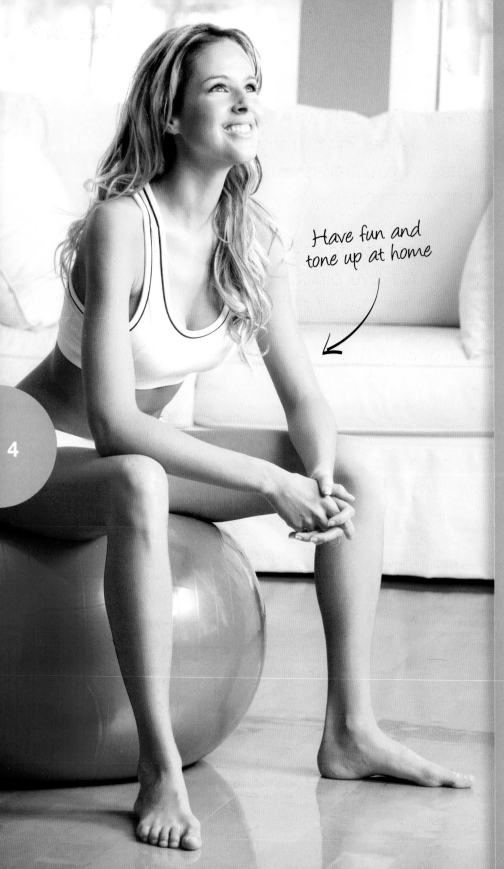

Have fun and tone up at home

4

Clothing credits

COVER
Women's VRV Reversible Bra
£18 | www.adidas.com
Verve Curve Shorts
£33 | www.noballs.co.uk

WARM UP
Training Top
£28 | www.adidas.com
Adilibria Leggings
£37 | www.adidas.com
Arianna II Trainers
£42 | www.adidas.com
Warrior Mat
£17.50 | www.yogamad.com

MAIN WORKOUT
Crop Top (underneath)
£18 | www.adidas.com
Synergy Button Boxback
£45 | www.casall.com
¾ Leggings
£20 | www.adidas.com
Adizero TR Trainers
£65 | www.adidas.com
Manduka Ekolite Mat
£45 | www.yogamatters.com

FAT BURNER
Leo Tank
£33 | www.noballs.co.uk
Synergy Shorts
£39.95 | www.cassall.com
Adizero TR Trainers
£65 | www.adidas.com
Manduka Eko Mat
£60 | www.yogamatters.com

COOL DOWN
All Sport Bra
£28 | www.sweatybetty.com
Ejecta Vest
£48 | www.sweatybetty.com
Supplex Cropped Pant
£42 | www.noballs.co.uk
Warrior Mat
£17.50 | www.yogamad.com

YOGA WORKOUT
Layered Top
£45 | www.fromclothing.com
Organic Cotton Crop Top
£28 | www.fromclothing.com
Organic Cotton ¾ Leggings
£45 | www.fromclothing.com
Manduka Ekolite Mat
£45 | www.yogamatters.com

OPENERS
Crop Top
£18 | www.adidas.com
Verve Curve Shorts
£33 | www.noballs.co.uk
Wide Neck Organic Cotton Sweat
£65 | www.fromclothing.com

EQUIPMENT
All from Physical Company
www.physicalcompany.co.uk

Welcome to *Women's Fitness' Tone Up At Home*; your very own personal trainer in your front room! Exercising at home means you'll always find time to fit in a session, you can wear what you like and it's free! What more could you ask for?

This book will tone you from top to toe in as little as 10 minutes, so whether it's bye-bye bingo wings, or hello flat tummy, you'll be feeling gorgeous in no time.

It doesn't take much to get started, simply find your favourite music and workout gear, warm up and then get toning!

Enjoy

Joanna

5

Editor Joanna Knight
Sub-Editor Charlotte Cox
Art Director Matt Reynolds
Editorial Assistant Amanda Khouv
Personal Trainer
Kristoph Thompson
Contributors Dave Fletcher,
Louise Pyne, Kristoph Thompson
Photography Simon Taylor (cover);
Danny Bird; Hugh Threlfall;
Giulia Di Cesare; Shutterstock
Cover Model Nikki Lupton, MOT
Models, www.motmodel.com
Model Lindsay Jay, W Athletic,
www.wathletic.com

**Digital Production
Manager** Nicky Baker
**Management MagBook
Publisher** Dharmesh Mistry
Operations Director Robin Ryan

Advertising Manager Katie Wood
MD of Advertising
Julian Lloyd-Evans
Newstrade Director David Barker
Chief Operating Officer
Brett Reynolds
Group Finance Director
Ian Leggett
Chief Executive James Tye
Chairman Felix Dennis

MAGBOOK

The MagBook brand is a
trademark of Dennis Publishing
Ltd. 30 Cleveland St, London
W1T 4JD. Company registered
in England. All material © Dennis
Publishing Ltd, licensed by Felden
2011, and may not be reproduced
in whole or part without the

consent of the publishers. *Tone
Up At Home* ISBN 1781060045.
Licensing & Syndication
To license this product please
contact Hannah Heagney on
+44 (0) 20 7907 6134 or email
hannah_heagney@dennis.co.uk
To syndicate content from
this product please contact
Anj Dosaj Halai on +44 (0)
20 7907 6132 or email anj_
dosaj-halai@dennis. co.uk

Liability
While every care was taken during
the production of this MagBook,
the publishers cannot be held
responsible for the accuracy of the
information or any consequence
arising from it. Dennis Publishing
takes no responsibility for the

companies advertising in this
MagBook. The paper used within
this MagBook is produced from
sustainable fibre, manufactured
by mills with a valid chain of
custody. Printed at BGPrint Ltd.

**Always check with your GP
before commencing an exercise
programme, especially if you
have been inactive for a long
period of time. Those with a
history of high blood pressure
or heart disease should obtain
medical clearance before
undertaking any activity.**

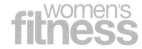

contents

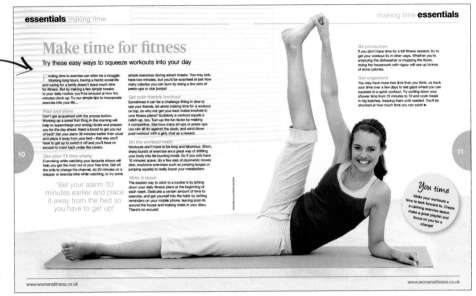

6

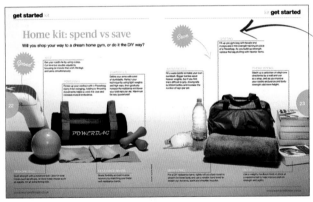

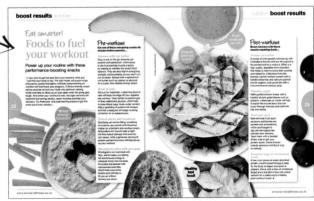

Contents

Exercise

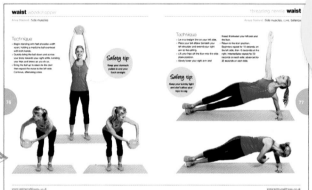

Toned in 10
Each of our fat-blasting
workouts can be
completed in just 10
minutes. Wow!

7

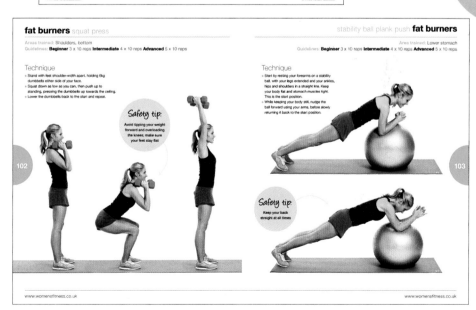

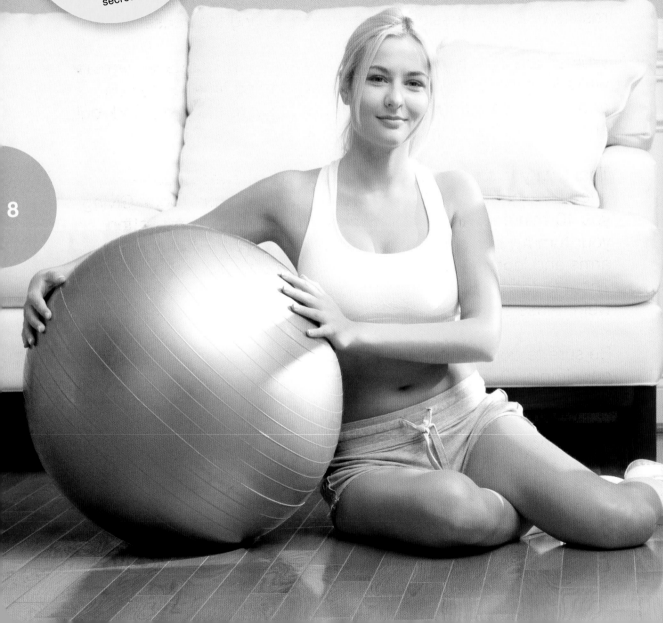

Shape up!

Getting fit and slimming down can seem scary. But don't worry! This book has all you need to know, from diet advice to fat-burning secrets.

Welcome

To *Women's Fitness' Tone Up At Home!* Here you can get the results of a gym session, without even leaving the house...

Women are always trying to squeeze more into our days, whether we're juggling a job with kids, or trying to find time for friends and family. So grabbing a spare hour to get to the gym, work out and then get home can be a mean feat.

That's why this home guide gives you short, sweet, super-effective workouts that get you fit in your own front room. Giving you 10-minute plans for every body part, this book will flatten your tummy, lift your bum, whittle your waist and shape your arms and legs, giving you the body you've always wanted. There's also a special fat-burning blast that *really* ups the weight-loss ante.

Be sure to complement your toning with our simple 10- and 20-minute cardio plans to really torch the calories.

'This guide has short, sweet, super-effective workouts that get you fit in your own front room!'

Stretching your newly honed body is important too, so breathe deep and relax with our favourite yoga poses. They'll do wonders for the inner – and slimmer – you!

So what are you waiting for? It's time to get toned – at home!

9

Make time for fitness

Try these easy ways to squeeze workouts into your day

Finding time to exercise can often be a struggle. Working long hours, having a hectic social life and caring for a family doesn't leave much time for fitness. But by making a few simple tweaks to your daily routine, you'll be amazed at how the minutes clock up. Try our simple tips to incorporate exercise into your life…

Rise and shine

Don't get acquainted with the snooze button. Working up a sweat first thing in the morning will help to supercharge your energy levels and prepare you for the day ahead. Need a boost to get you out of bed? Set your alarm 30 minutes earlier than usual and place it away from your bed – that way you'll have to get up to switch it off and you'll have no excuse to crawl back under the covers.

Use your TV time wisely

Exercising while watching your favourite shows will help you get the most out of your free time. Get off the sofa to change the channel, do 20 minutes on a stepper or exercise bike while watching, or try some simple exercises during advert breaks. You may only have two minutes, but you'd be surprised at just how many calories you can burn by doing a few sets of press-ups or star jumps!

Get your friends involved

Sometimes it can be a challenge fitting in time to see your friends, let alone making time for a workout on top, so why not get your best mates involved in your fitness plans? Suddenly a workout equals a catch-up, too. Turn up the fun factor by making it competitive. See how many sit-ups or press-ups you can all do against the clock; and wind down post-workout with a girly chat as a reward.

Do the workout math

Workouts don't have to be long and laborious. Short, sharp bursts of exercise are a great way of shifting your body into fat-burning mode. So if you only have 10 minutes spare, do a few sets of plyometric moves (fast, explosive exercises such as jumping lunges or jumping squats) to really boost your metabolism.

Write it down

The easiest way to stick to a routine is by jotting down your daily fitness plans at the beginning of each week. Dedicate a certain amount of time to exercise, and get yourself into the habit by setting reminders on your mobile phone, leaving post-its around the house and making notes in your diary. There's no excuse!

> 'Set your alarm 30 minutes earlier and place it away from the bed so you have to get up!'

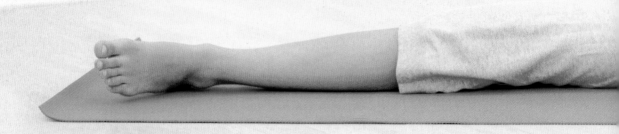

Be productive

If you don't have time for a full fitness session, try to get your workout fix in other ways. Whether you're emptying the dishwasher or mopping the floors, doing the housework with vigour will use up tonnes of extra calories.

Get organised

You may have more free time than you think, so track your time over a few days to see gaps where you can squeeze in a quick workout. Try cutting down your shower time from 15 minutes to 10 and cook meals in big batches, freezing them until needed. You'll be shocked at how much time you can save! ⓦ

11

You time

Make your workouts a time to look forward to. Create a calming exercise space, make a great playlist and focus on you for a change!

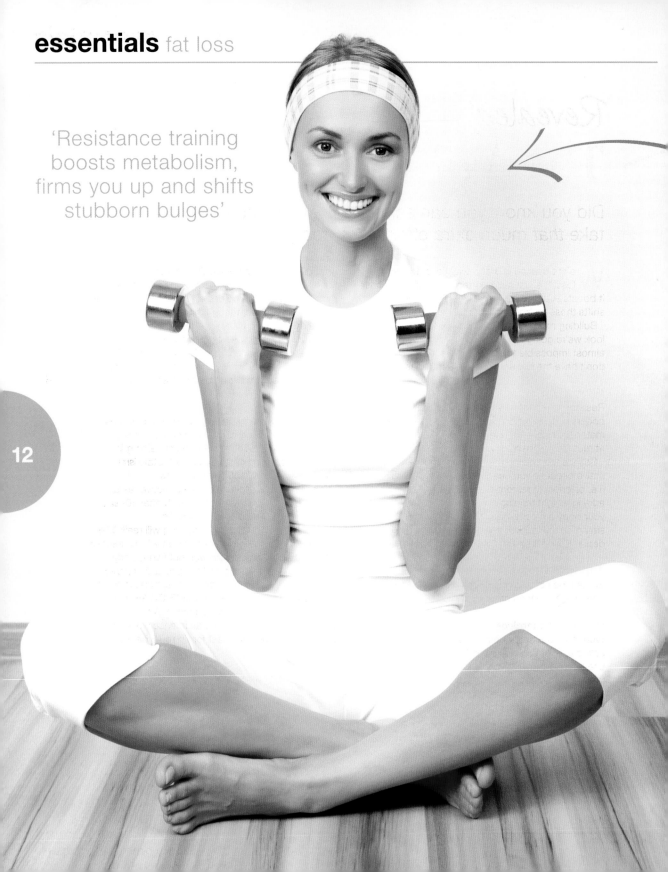

'Resistance training boosts metabolism, firms you up and shifts stubborn bulges'

12

Revealed!
The *real* secret to fat loss

Did you know you can shift fat for good, and it doesn't take *that* much extra effort? Yes, really!

Weight training is a one-way ticket to weight loss. It's just as important as cardio, because it boosts your metabolism, firms you up all over and shifts those stubborn bulges.

Building muscle doesn't mean bulk – that's not the look we're going for! However hard women train, it's almost impossible to end up like Arnie, because we don't have the hormones to build muscles like that.

Why more muscle = less fat

Resistance work (weight or body-weight training) boosts your lean muscle mass and raises your basal metabolic rate – the rate at which you burn calories at rest, doing absolutely nothing!

Resistance training makes you more metabolically active because you need to burn more energy (i.e. calories) to restore muscles you've used. By adding weight training to your workouts you'll make your body a calorie-burning machine (even while sitting on the sofa) *and* you'll help prevent bone degenerating diseases and heart disease. Bonus!

Top fat-burning techniques

Some types of exercise boost your fat-burning potential more than others:

Compound exercises

Working more than one muscle group at a time is called a 'compound exercise'. These exercises use as many muscles as possible to really boost the calorie burn. The exercises in this book target specific body parts, but most work more than one muscle group at a time.

Fast-twitch exercises

Our muscle fibres are split into two types: slow twitch and fast twitch. It's your fast-twitch fibres that really hold the fat-burning power. They contract quickly, fuelled by glycogen (stored sugar in the body) and the energy-carrying molecule ATP; and they provide strength and speed, though they also fatigue more quickly. Slow-twitch fibres, on the other hand, contract slowly and use oxygen as their primary energy source. Weights, sprints and circuits will stimulate your fast-twitch fibres, whereas aerobic exercise will set your slow-twitch muscles to work.

But what about cardio?

Cardio work certainly helps you to burn off fat, but there are smart ways to train so you don't have to slog it out for hours. Unless you're training for a distance event, running at a steady state isn't making the most of your workout time!

Short, sharp bursts mean more effective results in less time; so the plans in this book offer 10- and 20-minute intervals of at-home cardio.

Varying the intensity of your training will really blast the fat, too. Alternate between more and less intense intervals during your cardio workout (e.g. steady running and sprints) to boost fat loss and improve your stamina and endurance. What's more, interval training like this will increase your EPOC (excess post-oxygen energy consumption), which is your body's need to burn fat after an intense workout. The flab-fighting effects last for up to 48 hours!

Get the perfect mix

To really blast the fat, combine the cardio plans with the muscle toning workouts, all in the comfort of your own home. And if you feel like a serious challenge, turn to page 101 for the ultimate fat-burning workout. But be warned, it uses slightly heavier weights and is *not* for the faint hearted! ◪

Mix it up

Don't let your body get used to your exercise plan, keep it guessing with new moves!

13

Push yourself!
Be your own personal trainer

Follow these stay-on-track strategies to make sure you don't lose your willpower

206
minus 88% of your age
Is how to work out your max heart rate. If you're 30, 88% of your age is 26.4; and 206 - 26.4 = 179.6. So, your max is 180 beats per minute (bpm). You should work out at 60% of this, which is 108 bpm.

Splashing out on a personal trainer can be effective, but expensive. Save your money and empower yourself with these fail-safe fitness rules...

Rule 1: Set yourself goals
An important part of a PT's job is to map out a plan to help you reach your target. Set your own exercise goals, whether it's doing your home workout three times a week, upping the number of squats you can do or signing yourself up to an event. Having a goal will help to keep you focused.

Rule 2: Mix it up
Personal trainers tend to mix up exercises to keep workouts fresh and exciting. If you do the same moves day in, day out, you'll soon stop seeing results and boredom will set in. Keep your workouts interesting by pushing yourself as hard as you can and varying the moves – for example, if you've mastered the plank, try a one-legged version.

Rule 3: Reap the rewards
It's important to set fitness goals, but, as any good PT will tell you, it's also important to reward yourself when you achieve them. When you reach a milestone, treat yourself with a new outfit or spoil yourself with a pampering session at your local spa.

Rule 4: Get kitted out
Investing in some new workout kit is the best way to kick-start fitness, because you're more likely to stick to a routine if you feel good about yourself. Shop around for comfy clothing that fits you properly. A supportive sports bra, sweat-wicking vest top, sporty leggings and a good pair of cross-training shoes should be top of your kit list.

Rule 5: Take your measurements
Monitoring your progress is a great way to power up your workouts. Before you begin your exercise plan, get yourself a tape measure and record your vital stats, be sure to keep it handy to check out how many inches you're losing.

14

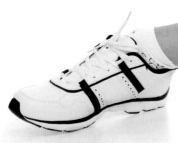

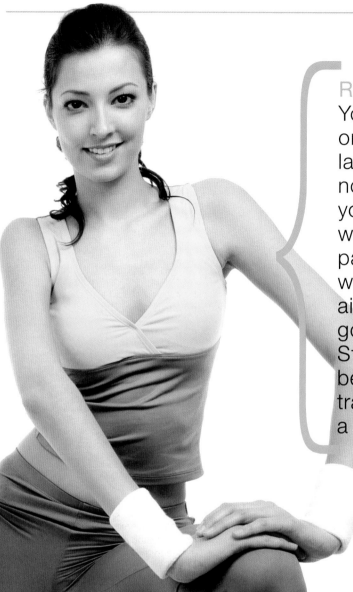

Rule 6: Have a plan

You wouldn't cancel on your trainer at the last minute, so there's no excuse to cancel on yourself! Think of your workout as an integral part of your working week. Write down your aims and how you're going to achieve them. Starting small is the best way to stay on track, so take exercise a little at a time.

Rule 7: *Raise your heart rate*

Pushing yourself to your limits can have a dramatic effect on results. Using a heart rate monitor helps you do this by showing a continuous reading of how hard you're working. To put your body into fat-burning mode, you should be working at no less than 60 per cent of your maximum heart rate – the fastest rate your heart will beat per minute. You can work out your maximum heart rate using the calculation at the top of the page. ◼

You wouldn't cancel on your trainer at the last minute, so there's no excuse to cancel on yourself!

It's so easy!
How to get started

It's time to get in to gear and get in shape!
Here's how to use this book

Before you start, check your form with our safety tips on page 20. Working out correctly will not only prevent injuries, it'll help you get the best results. Always warm up, too – from page 33 there are four essential moves to get your blood flowing and your joints and muscles ready.

Go for the burn
Cardio exercise is a great calorie burner, but research proves that interval training (a session that alternates spurts of moderate and high intensity exercise, e.g. alternating jogging and sprinting) is far better than steady-state cardio like a 30-minute jog. So, we've devised four super-effective cardio plans you can do at home, in just 10 or 20 minutes, from page 38.

Choose skipping, dancing, running on the spot or jumping, pop on some music and follow the plan. You'll work up a sweat and get much more from the workout than a fixed intensity one. This really is the way to train!

Tone up in time
You'll only lose weight if you combine cardio with toning exercises, so this book brings you the 10 best exercises for each body part. You'll be able to trim your tum, lift your bum, slim your waist and sculpt your legs and arms, all in just 10 minutes each!

Whether you have 10, 20 or 30 minutes, you can choose the workout for you. Mix and match from different body parts if time is short, or go for a total body blast if you have more time. There's also a fat-burning special on page 101, featuring the ultimate exercises to get you super results, super quick.

Know your level
To get the best results, first determine your finess level, then follow the guidelines on page 32 for either beginner, intermediate or advanced exercisers.

You're a **beginner** if you are new to exercise; you're an **intermediate** if you exercise two to three times a week; and you're an **advanced** exerciser if you work out four to five times a week.

Follow the cardio and toning plans for your level and use the expert nutritional advice to get your perfect body in no time!

Stretch it out
Stretching and relaxing is key to working out. Our yoga moves on page 111 will help you lengthen and strengthen while quietening the mind. The cool-down on page 121 will mean that you are ready for your next workout in better shape than you were before.

16

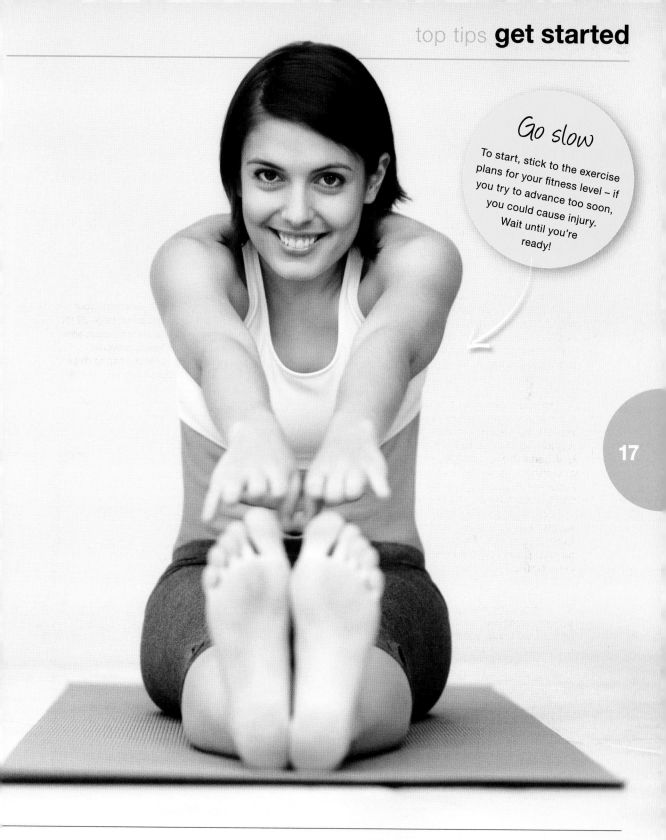

Go slow

To start, stick to the exercise plans for your fitness level – if you try to advance too soon, you could cause injury. Wait until you're ready!

17

Week 1

MONDAY

TUESDAY

WEDNESDAY

THURSDAY

FRIDAY

SATURDAY

SUNDAY

Week 2

MONDAY

TUESDAY

WEDNESDAY

THURSDAY

FRIDAY

SATURDAY

SUNDAY

18

Your 4-week plan

To stay on track, simply write down your workout plan for the days and weeks ahead. Then stick to it!

Week 3

MONDAY

TUESDAY

WEDNESDAY

THURSDAY

FRIDAY

SATURDAY

SUNDAY

Week 4

MONDAY

TUESDAY

WEDNESDAY

THURSDAY

FRIDAY

SATURDAY

SUNDAY

19

Tip: Copy this so you can use it again and again!

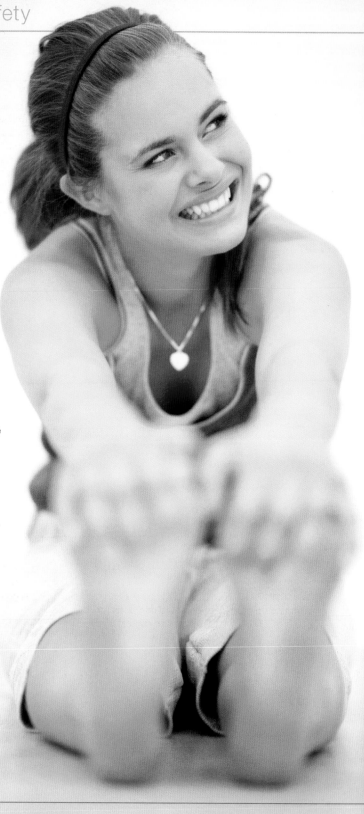

How to...
Have the perfect workout

Avoid injury and stay safe with these top tips

It's easy to overdo things in the first couple of weeks of a new fitness regime. You're bubbling over with enthusiasm and itching to shift those inches – but it's important to start slowly and listen to your body. You'll need to push yourself to see results, but don't try to do too much too soon. Spread your workouts throughout the week to allow for rest and recovery between sessions.

Listen to your body
Pay attention to any feedback your body gives you. Stop exercising if you experience pain or feel light headed; and any sharp pain during exercise is a sign that something is wrong. If this happens, stop exercising immediately. If you are still experiencing pain 48 hours later, it might be worth seeing a doctor or physio.

Mild soreness and aching muscles are to be expected in the days after your initial workouts. But don't panic, and don't let it put you off! Aches should ease during exercise and as you become more accustomed to your fitness programme.

Hydration

Drink water at regular intervals to prevent dehydration. When exercising, you can easily lose a litre of fluid in sweat each hour. Being even mildly dehydrated will impair your ability to exercise and stay cool, placing extra stress on the body. To prevent dehydration, keep a bottle of water to hand and take sips every 15-20 minutes.

lubricating fluid to better cover the inside of the joints, acting much like oil in a car engine to help them move easily.

Finish the warm-up with stretches for the major muscles of the upper and lower body, holding each for 10 seconds. Stretching lengthens the muscles in preparation for exercise and reduces the chances of pulls or tears.

Posture and technique

Using the correct technique when exercising helps to boost the benefits and reduce your risk of injury. Regardless of the type of activity, there are a number of postural tips to follow:

1. Keep your stomach pulled in and stomach muscles engaged to support your back
Activating your abs and core creates a protective corset around your torso, which helps to prevent lower back pain and injury.

2. Straighten, but don't lock, your joints
Forcibly locking your joints increases the risk of a sprain or strain. Smoothly straighten your arms and legs, stopping just short of locking. Keep your knees soft when standing to allow your legs to absorb any downward forces.

3. Land softly on the balls of your feet when running, jumping and skipping
A hard landing means the impact isn't efficiently absorbed by your hips, knees and ankles, and can result in an injury. Your landings should be fairly quiet, with the joints of the lower body slightly bent to better absorb the landing forces.

Cooling down

Finish each workout with a few minutes of gentle activity, such as jogging on the spot, gradually reducing the pace to a march and then a walk. Finish by doing the cool-down stretches, which start on page 121. Your cool-down is vital as it is the first stage in the recovery process and will help you to recover and adapt more quickly. ◼

Warming up

Warming up prepares your mind and body for exercise, and helps to reduce the risk of injury and the likelihood of sore muscles after your workout.

Start your warm-up with a few minutes of light activity, such as marching or jogging on the spot, to raise your heart rate and boost the flow of blood around the body.

Next, mobilise your joints by doing the exercises on pages 33 to 37. These moves will help the body's

Get it right!

Fewer exercises done with correct form are more effective than many done inaccurately

21

Home kit: spend vs save

Will you shop your way to a dream home gym, or do it the DIY way?

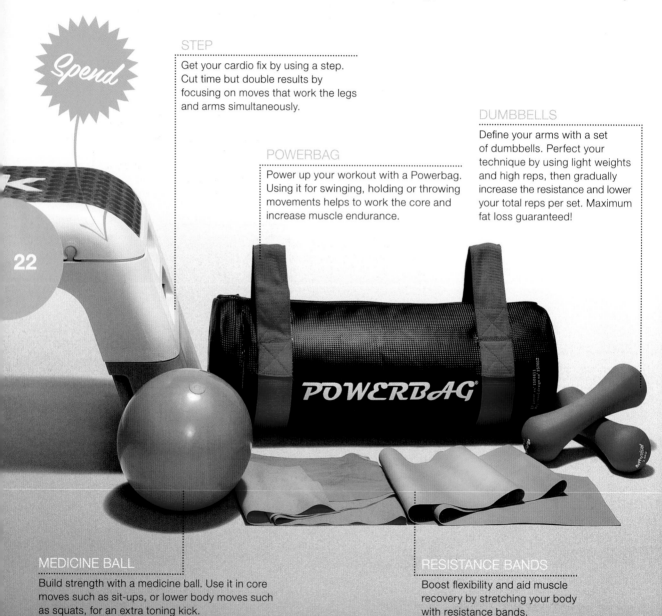

Spend

STEP

Get your cardio fix by using a step. Cut time but double results by focusing on moves that work the legs and arms simultaneously.

POWERBAG

Power up your workout with a Powerbag. Using it for swinging, holding or throwing movements helps to work the core and increase muscle endurance.

DUMBBELLS

Define your arms with a set of dumbbells. Perfect your technique by using light weights and high reps, then gradually increase the resistance and lower your total reps per set. Maximum fat loss guaranteed!

22

MEDICINE BALL

Build strength with a medicine ball. Use it in core moves such as sit-ups, or lower body moves such as squats, for an extra toning kick.

RESISTANCE BANDS

Boost flexibility and aid muscle recovery by stretching your body with resistance bands.

Save

GYM BAG
Fill up you gym bag with towels and incorporate it into strength training in place of a Powerbag. As you build up strength, replace the bag stuffing with heavier items.

WATER BOTTLE
Fill a water bottle to make your own dumbbell. Bigger bottles equal heavier weights, but if you find them difficult to grip, downgrade to 500ml bottles and increase the number of reps per set.

PHONE BOOKS
Stack up a selection of telephone directories by a wall and use as a step, and as you improve your cardio endurance and body strength add more height.

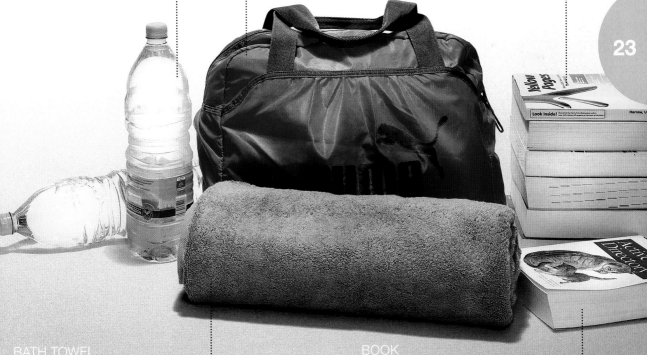

23

BATH TOWEL
For a DIY resistance band, tightly roll up a bath towel to stretch the lower body and use a smaller hand towel to stretch out the arms, back and shoulder muscles.

BOOK
Use a weighty hardback book in place of a medicine ball to help improve posture, strength and agility.

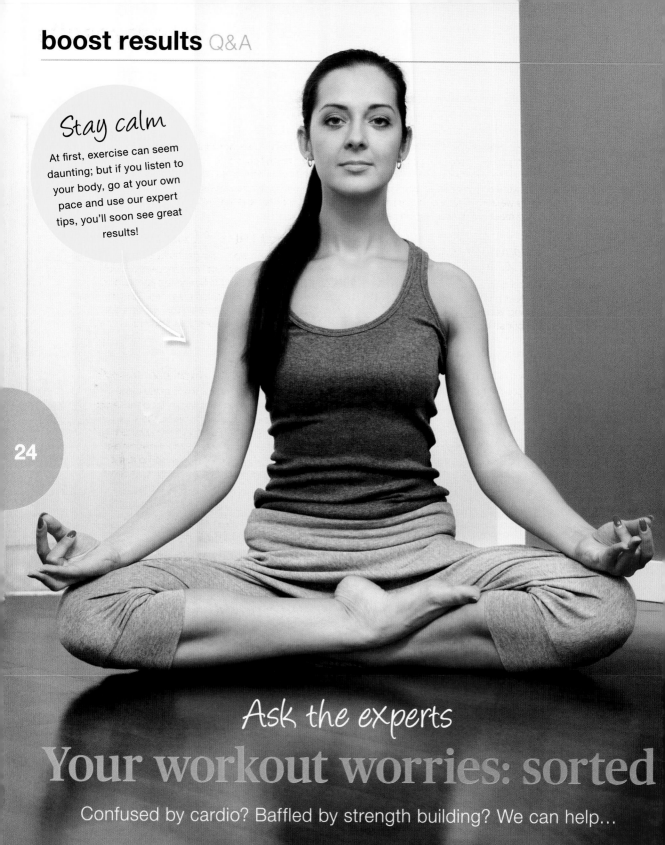

Stay calm

At first, exercise can seem daunting; but if you listen to your body, go at your own pace and use our expert tips, you'll soon see great results!

24

Ask the experts

Your workout worries: sorted

Confused by cardio? Baffled by strength building? We can help...

Whether you're wondering when's the best time of the day to work out, what's the most effective way to burn fat, or whether weary muscles are a sign of hard work or something more serious, then fear not. Here we solve your workout dilemmas to help you get the most out of every single session.

Q Should I do my strength or cardio exercises first?

Since you are going to be fatigued towards the end of your workout, your performance will be affected in whichever training you choose to do second. However, doing your strength training before your cardio will have a less noticeable impact on your cardio performance, and may increase the amount of fat you burn. Conversely, doing your cardio before strength may lower your capabilities in the strength training exercises and limit your results.

Q Will I get bulky if I work out?

It's very difficult for women to get bulky through exercise. Building muscle not only requires *a lot* of weight training, but also the hormone testosterone, which is much lower in women than men. Rather than causing muscles to swell in size, working out will give you a more toned physique and reduce levels of stored body fat.

Q Should I exercise when I'm aching?

It's normal to experience soreness in the days following a workout, and continuing to exercise can actually help the recovery process. Make sure you warm up thoroughly to loosen stiff muscles and get blood flowing around the body, and the soreness should reduce when you start your workout. If it doesn't, or it gets worse, stop exercising and rest that part of the body for a couple of days.

Q When is the best time of day to exercise and why?

The best time is the one that fits in best with your plans, and this can change from one day to the next. Some people may like to start the day with a workout, others prefer to exercise later in the day. Experiment with different workout times, deciding which one(s) work best for you.

Q How high does my heart rate have to be to burn fat?

An easy sum can help you work out your maximum heart rate: subtract 88% of your age from 206 (see page 15). Exercise intensity tends to be expressed as a percentage of your maximum heart rate. Exercising at 60 per cent will burn fat and increase your fitness levels. Exercising at a lower intensity requires less energy and burns fewer calories.

Q Can I target specific parts of my body?

Specific exercises target certain muscles and, although it's not possible to reduce fat levels specifically in these areas, it *is* possible to tone the muscles. Exercises such as lunges tone the thighs and bottom, while crunches target the stomach and push-ups work the chest and shoulders. ◼

25

How to...
Fight fat with food

Follow these strategies to supercharge your slim-down

While exercise is an essential part of any slim-down plan, eating the right foods is a surefire way to see results. Feeding your body with the right nutrients will help to put it into fat-burning mode, naturally boosting your metabolism and melting away excess pounds. Follow these golden rules for fast results:

Fill up on fibre
Fibre keeps you fuller for longer by delaying the rate at which food leaves the stomach, which helps to stabilise blood sugar levels. Load up on fruit and veg, legumes, oats and wholegrains to get your daily quota and, for an extra metabolism boost, add spices such as turmeric and chilli to meals.

Drink enough water
When you are dehydrated, fat cells become harder to break down, which causes your body to cling on to the excess pounds. What's more, thirst can often be confused with hunger – so, before you reach for food, drink a glass of water instead. You should aim for around two to three litres per day.

Add protein
Make sure protein is factored into every meal. Your body needs this macronutrient to maintain lean muscle, so it's an essential part of recovery from exercise. Combining protein with carbohydrates will also help to curb hunger. Good choices include beans, lentils, tofu, fish and lean meat (such as chicken or turkey) served with wholegrains like brown rice.

Avoid sugar
Sugar raises your levels of the blood-regulating hormone insulin, and is one of the main culprits of fat storage. It's also associated with obesity and long-term conditions like diabetes.

Go natural
A lot of supermarket produce is packed with artificial chemicals, hormones and preservatives. Your body doesn't know how to process these nasties, so instead of getting rid of them, it stores them in fat cells. Try to buy organic wherever possible and always read the ingredient list of any given food.

Limit fizzy drinks, alcohol and processed foods; sweeten foods naturally with dark-skinned fruits, appetite-curbing cinnamon or a spoonful of honey.

Eat fat to lose fat
Don't be scared of fat! The good fats found in nuts, avocados, cold pressed oils and oily fish like salmon and mackerel promote weight loss, keep you

Safety tip:
To lose weight safely, slow and steady is the key. Aim for around 1-2lbs a week.

26

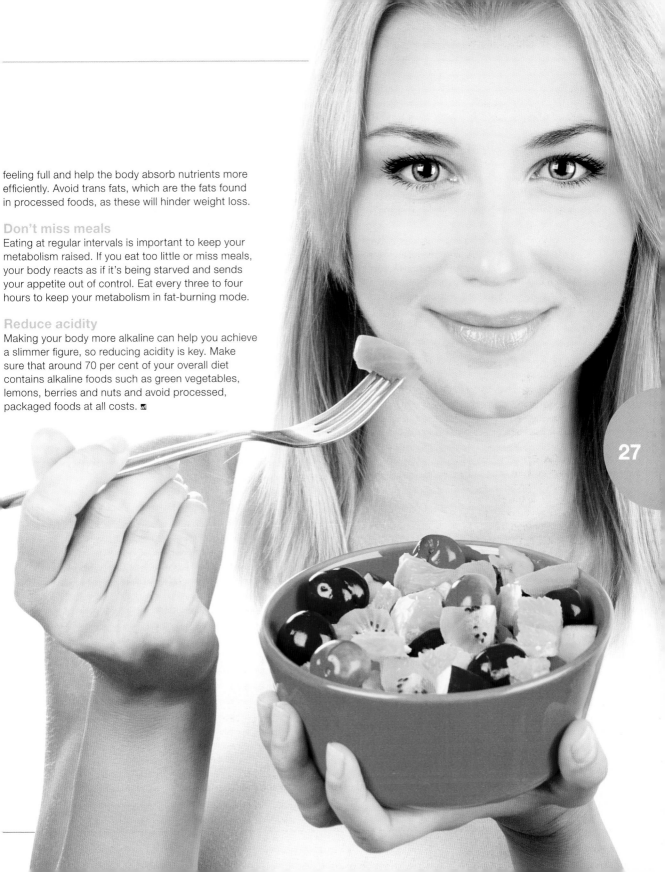

feeling full and help the body absorb nutrients more efficiently. Avoid trans fats, which are the fats found in processed foods, as these will hinder weight loss.

Don't miss meals

Eating at regular intervals is important to keep your metabolism raised. If you eat too little or miss meals, your body reacts as if it's being starved and sends your appetite out of control. Eat every three to four hours to keep your metabolism in fat-burning mode.

Reduce acidity

Making your body more alkaline can help you achieve a slimmer figure, so reducing acidity is key. Make sure that around 70 per cent of your overall diet contains alkaline foods such as green vegetables, lemons, berries and nuts and avoid processed, packaged foods at all costs. ▨

Eat smarter!
Foods to fuel your workout

Power up your routine with these performance-boosting snacks

If you want to get the best from your workout, what you put into your body is key. The right foods will supercharge endurance, speed and agility; whereas compromising on nutrition will hold back your progress. A fitness-friendly snack before exercise will put your body into optimum training mode and help to keep you at your peak when the going gets tough. And when your workout is over, the right nutrients will replenish lost energy stores, repair muscles and help your recovery. Try these pre- and post-training snacks to get the most out of your session…

Great energy booster!

28

Pre-workout
Eat one of these energising snacks 45 minutes before exercise…

Banana with nut butter
Easy to eat on the go, bananas are packed with potassium, which plays a role in preventing muscle cramps by helping to maintain the body's fluid balance. They are also high in energising complex carbohydrates, so you won't run out of steam. Spread with a spoonful of nut butter (such as cashew or almond) for a super slow-release energy snack.

Bowl of oats
Not just for breakfast, a steaming bowl of oats will keep the edge off your appetite pre-workout. Oats contain a special type of fibre called beta-glucans, which help to keep blood sugar levels under control. Add a sprinkling of protein-rich linseed and half a teaspoon of hunger-curbing cinnamon for an added boost.

Carrot sticks and houmous
Satisfying yet not too filling, munching on crunchy raw carrots with houmous makes for a fantastic pre-workout snack. Antioxidant-rich carrots help to fight the free radical damage that exercise can cause, while a generous serving of protein-packed houmous will help power up your workout.

Wholegrain pitta with avocado
Wholegrains are crammed with fibre, which keeps you feeling full and ensures energy is released slowly into the body. Avocados are packed with monounsaturated fats, which keep your joints flexible and will help to fill you up without slowing you down.

Post workout reviver!

Protein packed snack!

Healthy fast food!

Post-workout

Boost recovery with these muscle-repairing foods...

Protein smoothie

A scoop of whey protein whizzed up with a handful of berries and low fat yoghurt is the perfect end to a workout. Whey is a high quality, digestible form of protein that helps to feed muscles after exercise and makes for a fabulous immunity booster. Up the nutrient content with a handful of berries and calcium-packed low fat yoghurt, and you're left with a convenient post-workout treat.

Chicken salad

Half a grilled chicken breast with a handful of dark green leaves such as spinach, watercress or rocket will help to repair the muscle tears that can occur through exercise and replenish lost iron stores.

Fruit and nuts

Dark-skinned fruits such as plums and berries are packed with antioxidants, which are thought to zap cell-damaging free radicals after exercise. Team them with a handful of raw nuts to get your protein quota. Good choices include selenium-rich Brazil nuts or walnuts.

Poached egg on wholemeal toast

A low-cost source of easily absorbed protein, a softly poached egg is easy for the body to digest and quick to prepare. Serve with a slice of wholemeal bread and a handful of iron-rich wilted spinach for a satisfying but healthy post-workout snack. ⓦ

29

HAVE YOU GOT
WHAT IT TAKES TO

CHANGE?

Whether you are working towards your ideal physique in terms of appearance or whether you need your physique to deliver increased performance, you have a challenge on your hands.

Without maximizing each important component, you are likely to compromise or fail in your goals. When it comes to supplements, you might well need to change your views.

If you don't change your views, you may already have failed in your goals.

> **We've changed the industry standards of protein products for you.**

> **We've changed what value for money can mean to you.**

> **We've changed how products are formulated with you in mind.**

> **We've changed how products are produced providing you with both performance and health.**

> **We've changed the type of guarantee that you can expect.**

> **We're totally committed to make changes to your physique and health more achievable.**

Find out more about these changes at:

www.reflex-nutrition.com

 Please visit & join our Facebook page at Reflex Nutrition Ltd

 @ReflexNutrition

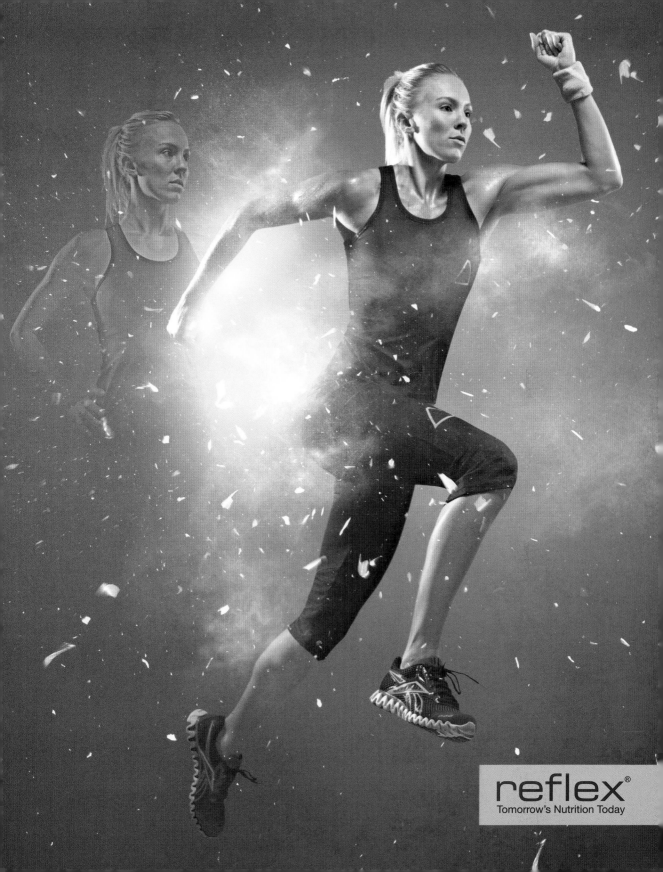

reflex®
Tomorrow's Nutrition Today

It is time to...
Get started!

Create your perfect workout using our easy guide

Getting fit at home is all about you, you, you. This is YOUR workout, so make every minute your own!

Warm up your body with the exercises on pages 32-37, then choose the body part you want to work and pick your intensity level from the guides below. Next, turn the page to your chosen workout and perform every exercise for a targeted 10-minute tone-up. Or, for a longer session, mix and match your 10-minute workouts to get the combination YOU want.

Combine these toning moves with the cardio plans on page 38 to get the ultimate fat-burning results.

Beginners should aim for two workouts a week; intermediates should aim for three; and advanced should go for four.

Find your ideal weights

32

Toning guidelines:

Find the ideal timing for your fitness level:

Beginner
Do each exercise for 30 seconds, then rest for 30 seconds before moving on to the next exercise

Intermediate
Do each exercise for 40 seconds, then rest for 20 seconds before moving on to the next exercise

Advanced
Do each exercise for 50 seconds, then rest for 10 seconds before moving on to the next exercise

Important!

If you find any exercise too tough, do it for as long as you can while your form is perfect, then rest. Just be sure to keep challenging yourself in future sessions.

Weights guidelines:

Perform each toning exercise, using the right weights (where necessary) for your fitness level for each body part:

Tummy
Beginner: 2-5kg
Intermediate: 3-6kg
Advanced: 4-6kg

Bottom
Beginner: 3-8kg
Intermediate: 4-10kg
Advanced: 6-10kg

Waist
Beginners: 3-4kg

Intermediate: 3-5kg
Advanced: 4-6kg

Legs
Beginner: 5-10kg
Intermediate: 6-12kg
Advanced: 8-12kg

Arms
Beginners: 3-5kg
Intermediate: 4-6kg
Adavanced: 5-6kg

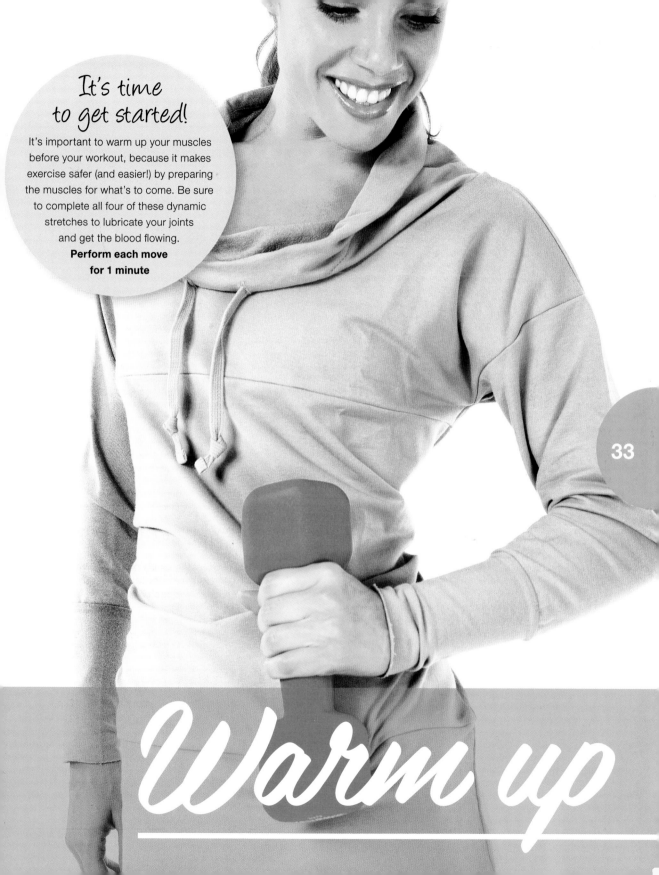

It's time to get started!

It's important to warm up your muscles before your workout, because it makes exercise safer (and easier!) by preparing the muscles for what's to come. Be sure to complete all four of these dynamic stretches to lubricate your joints and get the blood flowing. **Perform each move for 1 minute**

33

Warm up

warm up squat, reach and twist

Areas warmed up: Front and back of thighs, inner thighs, bottom, side muscles, middle of back

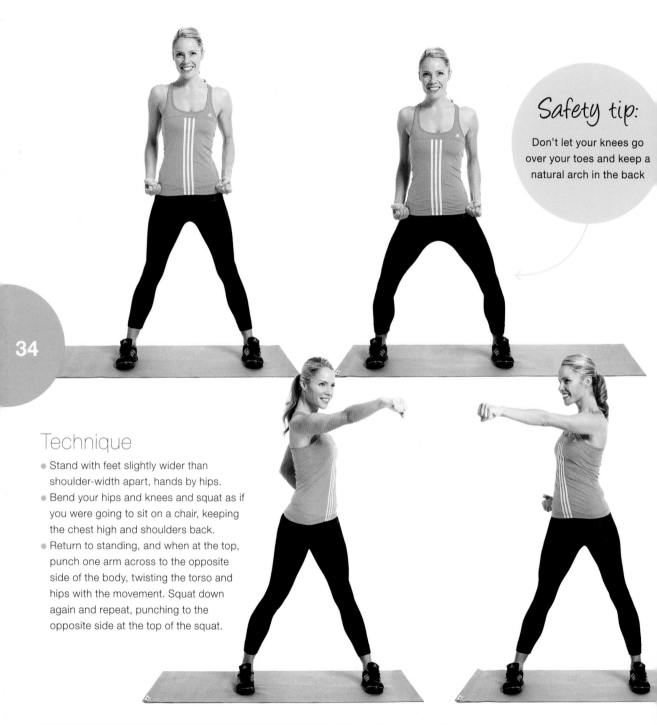

Safety tip:

Don't let your knees go over your toes and keep a natural arch in the back

Technique

- Stand with feet slightly wider than shoulder-width apart, hands by hips.
- Bend your hips and knees and squat as if you were going to sit on a chair, keeping the chest high and shoulders back.
- Return to standing, and when at the top, punch one arm across to the opposite side of the body, twisting the torso and hips with the movement. Squat down again and repeat, punching to the opposite side at the top of the squat.

Areas warmed up: Back of thighs, calves, bottom, hips

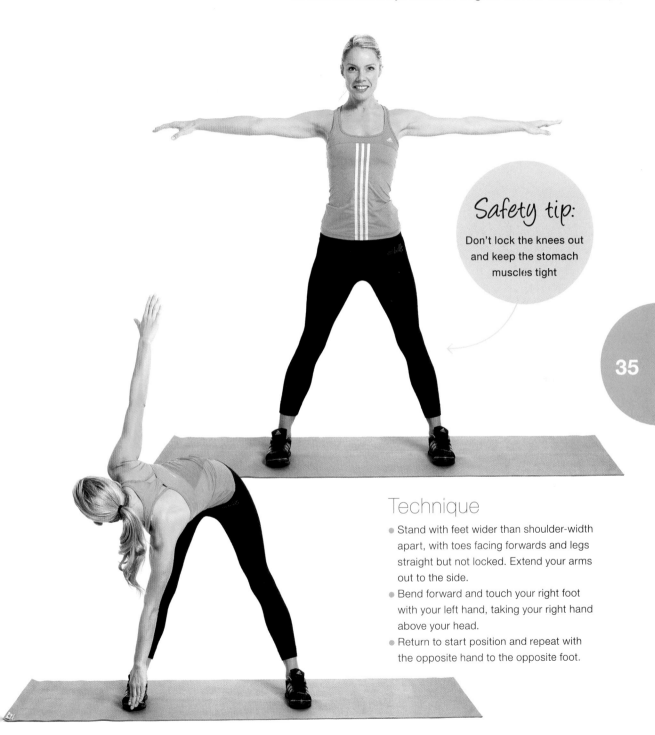

Safety tip:

Don't lock the knees out and keep the stomach muscles tight

35

Technique

- Stand with feet wider than shoulder-width apart, with toes facing forwards and legs straight but not locked. Extend your arms out to the side.
- Bend forward and touch your right foot with your left hand, taking your right hand above your head.
- Return to start position and repeat with the opposite hand to the opposite foot.

warm up hip circles

Areas warmed up: Hips, stomach

Technique

- Stand with feet slightly wider than shoulder-width apart with hands on hips.
- Circle your hips in a clockwise direction for 10 full circles, then repeat in the opposite direction. Repeat for one minute.

Safety tip:

Don't lock the knees out and keep the back straight

36

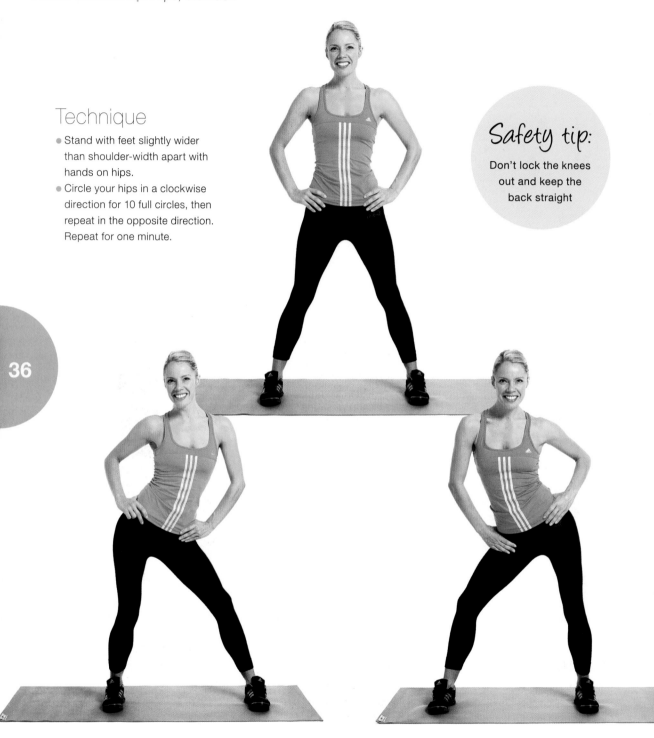

Areas warmed up: Shoulders, chest

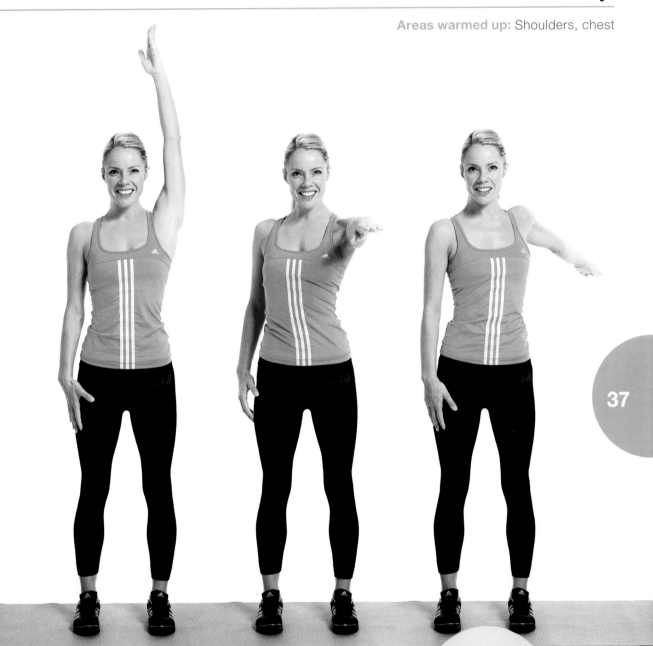

37

Technique

- Stand with feet hip-width apart, left arm extended straight up in the air.
- Circle the arm in a forwards direction for 15 seconds, and repeat with the right arm for 15 seconds. Then circle each arm in a backwards direction, both for 15 seconds.

Safety tip:

Keep the elbows soft and back straight

plans skipping

...he speed of your skips according to
...nsity required (see box, right).
...ftly on the balls of your feet, only
... as high as you need to allow the
... pass underneath you.

There's a cardio workout for everyone, so pick your favourite and start your four-week plan!
Measure your intensity based on a scale of 1-10. Level 10 is all-out effort, which you can't maintain for more than 30 seconds. Your breathing will be heavy and you should find it difficult to talk when working at this intensity. Level 1 is minimal effort, the equivalent of a slow walk, and your breathing should be normal. You should be able to comfortably maintain this level for an extended period.

20-minute workout

Beginner repeat twice a week

Week 1	Week 2	Week 3	Week 4
1 min level 4	1 min level 5	1 min level 6	1 min level 6
1 min level 5	1 min level 7	1 min level 8	1 min level 9
1 min level 6	1 min level 8	1 min level 6	1 min level 6
1 min level 8	1 min level 5	1 min level 6	1 min level 8
1 min level 6	1 min level 7	1 min level 6	1 min level 6
1 min level 8	1 min level 8	1 min level 8	1 min level 9
1 min level 6	1 min level 5	1 min level 6	1 min level 6
1 min level 7	1 min level 7	1 min level 9	1 min level 8
1 min level 9	1 min level 9	1 min level 6	1 min level 9
1 min level 6	1 min level 7	1 min level 9	1 min level 9

Intermediate repeat three times a week

Week 1	Week 2	Week 3	Week 4
1 min level 6	1 min level 6	1 min level 6	1 min level 7
1 min level 8	1 min level 9	1 min level 8	1 min level 9
1 min level 6	1 min level 6	1 min level 9	1 min level 8
1 min level 8	1 min level 8	1 min level 6	1 min level 7
1 min level 6	1 min level 6	1 min level 8	1 min level 8
1 min level 8	1 min level 8	1 min level 9	1 min level 9
1 min level 6	1 min level 6	1 min level 6	1 min level 8
1 min level 9	1 min level 9	1 min level 8	1 min level 7
1 min level 6	1 min level 6	1 min level 9	1 min level 9
1 min level 9	1 min level 6	1 min level 7	1 min level 7

Advanced repeat four times a week

Week 1	Week 2	Week 3	Week 4
1 min level 6	1 min level 7	1 min level 7	1 min level 7
1 min level 8	1 min level 9	1 min level 9	1 min level 9
1 min level 9	1 min level 8	1 min level 8	1 min level 8
1 min level 6	1 min level 7	1 min level 9	1 min level 8
1 min level 8	1 min level 8	1 min level 7	1 min level 9
1 min level 9	1 min level 9	1 min level 9	1 min level 9
1 min level 6	1 min level 8	1 min level 8	1 min level 7
1 min level 8	1 min level 7	1 min level 9	1 min level 9
1 min level 9	1 min level 9	1 min level 8	1 min level 8
1 min level 7	1 min level 7	1 min level 7	1 min level 9

Beginner repeat twice a week

Week 1	Week 2	Week 3	Week 4
2 mins level 4	2 mins level 5	2 mins level 6	2 mins level 6
1 min level 5	1 min level 7	2 mins level 8	2 mins level 8
2 mins level 6	2 mins level 6	2 mins level 6	2 mins level 6
1.5 mins level 8	1.5 mins level 8	1 min level 9	1 min level 9
2 mins level 6	2 mins level 6	2 mins level 6	2 mins level 7
1.5 mins level 8	1.5 mins level 8	1.5 mins level 8	2 mins level 8
1.5 mins level 7	1.5 mins level 8	2 mins level 6	2 mins level 6
1 min level 9	1 min level 9	1 min level 9	1 min level 9
2 mins level 6	2 mins level 7	1 min level 9	1 min level 7
1.5 mins level 7	1.5 mins level 8	2 mins level 6	2 mins level 7
2 mins level 6	2 mins level 6	1.5 mins level 8	1 min level 8

Intermediate repeat three times a week

Week 1	Week 2	Week 3	Week 4
2 mins level 6	2 mins level 6	2 mins level 6	2 mins level 7
1.5 mins level 8	1 min level 9	1.5 mins level 8	1 min level 9
2 mins level 6	2 mins level 6	1 min level 9	1.5 mins level 8
1.5 mins level 8	1.5 mins level 8	2 mins level 6	2 mins level 7
2 mins level 6	2 mins level 6	1.5 mins level 8	1.5 mins level 8
1.5 mins level 8	1 min level 9	1 min level 9	1 min level 9
2 mins level 6	2 mins level 6	2 mins level 6	1.5 mins level 8
1 min level 9	1 min level 9	1.5 mins level 8	2 mins level 7
2 mins level 6	2 mins level 6	1 min level 9	1 min level 9
1 min level 9	1 min level 9	2 mins level 7	2 mins level 7
2 mins level 7	2 mins level 7	1.5 mins level 8	1.5 mins level 8
1.5 mins level 8	1.5 mins level 8	2 mins level 7	1 min level 9
–	1 min level 9	1 min level 9	2 mins level 7

Advanced repeat four times a week

Week 1	Week 2	Week 3	Week 4
2 mins level 6	2 mins level 7	2 mins level 7	2 mins level 7
2 mins level 8	1 min level 9	1 min level 9	1 min level 9
1 min level 9	2 mins level 8	2 mins level 8	2 mins level 8
2 mins level 6	2 mins level 7	1 min level 9	1 min level 9
2 mins level 8	2 mins level 8	2 mins level 7	2 mins level 8
1 min level 9	1 min level 9	1 min level 9	1 min level 9
2 mins level 6	2 mins level 8	2 mins level 8	2 mins level 8
2 mins level 8	2 mins level 7	1 min level 9	1 min level 9
1 min level 9	1 min level 9	2 mins level 8	2 mins level 8
2 mins level 7	2 mins level 7	2 mins level 7	1 min level 9
1 min level 9	1 min level 9	1 min level 9	2 mins level 7
2 mins level 8	2 mins level 8	2 mins level 8	1 min level 9
–	–	1 min level 9	2 mins level 7

- Adjust the height and speed of your jumps according to the intensity required.
- Land softly, jumping again as soon as you can.

Key:
Stars = star jumps
SLH = single-leg hops

10-minute workout

Beginner repeat twice a week

Week 1	Week 2	Week 3	Week 4
1 min stars level 5	1 min stars level 5	1 min SLH level 6	1 min SLH level 6
1 min SLH level 6	1 min SLH level 7	1 min stars level 8	1 min SLH level 9
1 min stars level 7	1 min SLH level 8	1 min stars level 6	1 min SLH level 6
1 min stars level 6	1 min stars level 6	1 min SLH level 8	1 min stars level 8
1 min SLH level 6	1 min SLH level 7	1 min stars level 6	1 min SLH level 6
1 min SLH level 8	1 min SLH level 8	1 min stars level 8	1 min SLH level 9
1 min stars level 6	1 min stars level 5	1 min SLH level 6	1 min stars level 6
1 min SLH level 7	1 min SLH level 7	1 min SLH level 9	1 min stars level 8
1 min stars level 9	1 min stars level 9	1 min stars level 6	1 min SLH level 6
1 min stars level 6	1 min SLH level 7	1 min stars level 9	1 min SLH level 6

Beginner repeat twice a week

Week 1	Week 2	Week 3	Week 4
2 mins stars level 4	2 mins SLH level 5	2 mins SLH level 6	2 mins stars level 6
1 min SLH level 5	1 min stars level 7	2 mins stars level 8	2 mins SLH level 8
2 mins stars level 6	2 mins SLH level 6	2 mins SLH level 6	2 mins stars level 6
1.5 mins SLH level 8	1.5 mins stars level 8	1 min stars level 9	1 min SLH level 9
2 mins stars level 6	2 mins stars level 6	2 mins SLH level 6	2 mins SLH level 7
1.5 mins SLH level 8	1.5 mins SLH level 8	1.5 mins stars level 8	2 mins stars level 8
2 mins stars level 6	2 mins stars level 6	2 mins SLH level 6	2 mins SLH level 6
1.5 mins SLH level 7	1.5 mins SLH level 8	1 min stars level 9	1 min stars level 9
1 min stars level 9	1 min SLH level 9	2 mins SLH level 6	2 mins SLH level 7
2 mins SLH level 6	2 mins SLH level 7	1 min stars level 9	1 min stars level 9
1.5 mins SLH level 7	1.5 mins stars level 8	2 mins SLH level 6	2 mins SLH level 7
2 mins SLH level 6	2 mins stars level 6	1.5 mins stars level 8	1 min stars level 8

Intermediate repeat three times a week

Week 1	Week 2	Week 3	Week 4
1 min SLH level 6	1 min SLH level 6	1 min stars level 6	1 min stars level 7
1 min stars level 8	1 min stars level 9	1 min SLH level 8	1 min stars level 9
1 min SLH level 6	1 min SLH level 6	1 min stars level 9	1 min SLH level 8
1 min SLH level 8	1 min stars level 8	1 min stars level 6	1 min SLH level 7
1 min stars level 6	1 min stars level 6	1 min SLH level 8	1 min stars level 8
1 min stars level 8	1 min SLH level 9	1 min stars level 8	1 min stars level 9
1 min SLH level 6	1 min stars level 9	1 min stars level 6	1 min SLH level 8
1 min stars level 9	1 min stars level 9	1 min SLH level 8	1 min stars level 7
1 min SLH level 6	1 min stars level 6	1 min stars level 9	1 min SLH level 9
1 min SLH level 9	1 min SLH level 9	1 min SLH level 7	1 min stars level 7

Intermediate repeat three times a week

Week 1	Week 2	Week 3	Week 4
2 mins stars level 6	2 mins stars level 6	2 mins SLH level 6	2 mins stars level 7
1.5 mins SLH level 8	2 mins SLH level 9	1 min stars level 8	1 min SLH level 9
2 mins stars level 6	2 mins stars level 6	1 min SLH level 9	1.5 mins stars level 8
1.5 mins SLH level 8	1.5 mins SLH level 8	2 mins stars level 6	2 mins SLH level 7
2 mins stars level 6	2 mins stars level 6	1.5 mins SLH level 8	1.5 mins stars level 8
1.5 mins stars level 8	1 min SLH level 9	1 min stars level 9	1 min SLH level 9
2 mins SLH level 6	2 mins stars level 6	2 mins SLH level 6	1.5 mins SLH level 8
1 min stars level 9	1 min SLH level 9	1.5 mins stars level 8	2 mins SLH level 7
2 mins SLH level 6	2 mins stars level 6	1 min SLH level 9	1 min stars level 9
1 min stars level 9	1 min SLH level 9	2 mins stars level 7	2 mins SLH level 7
2 mins SLH level 7	2 mins stars level 7	1.5 mins SLH level 8	1.5 mins stars level 8
1.5 mins stars level 8	1.5 mins SLH level 8	2 mins stars level 7	1 min SLH level 9
–	–	1.5 mins stars level 8	2 mins stars level 7

Advanced repeat four times a week

Week 1	Week 2	Week 3	Week 4
1 min stars level 8	1 min SLH level 7	1 min stars level 7	1 min SLH level 7
1 min SLH level 8	1 min stars level 9	1 min SLH level 9	1 min stars level 9
1 min stars level 9	1 min SLH level 8	1 min stars level 8	1 min SLH level 8
1 min SLH level 6	1 min stars level 9	1 min stars level 7	1 min stars level 9
1 min stars level 8	1 min SLH level 8	1 min stars level 7	1 min SLH level 8
1 min SLH level 9	1 min stars level 9	1 min SLH level 9	1 min stars level 9
1 min stars level 6	1 min SLH level 8	1 min SLH level 8	1 min stars level 7
1 min stars level 8	1 min stars level 7	1 min stars level 9	1 min SLH level 9
1 min stars level 8	1 min SLH level 8	1 min stars level 9	1 min stars level 9
1 min stars level 9	1 min SLH level 9	1 min SLH level 8	1 min stars level 8

Advanced repeat four times a week

Week 1	Week 2	Week 3	Week 4
2 mins stars level 6	2 mins SLH level 7	2 mins stars level 7	2 mins stars level 7
2 mins SLH level 8	1 min stars level 9	1 min SLH level 9	1 min SLH level 9
1 min stars level 9	2 mins SLH level 8	2 mins stars level 8	2 mins stars level 8
2 mins SLH level 6	2 mins stars level 7	1 min SLH level 9	1 min SLH level 9
2 mins stars level 8	2 mins SLH level 8	2 mins stars level 7	2 mins stars level 8
1 min SLH level 9	1 min stars level 9	1 min SLH level 9	1 min SLH level 9
2 mins stars level 6	2 mins SLH level 8	2 mins stars level 8	2 mins stars level 7
2 mins SLH level 8	2 mins stars level 7	1 min SLH level 9	1 min SLH level 9
1 min stars level 9	1 min SLH level 9	2 mins stars level 8	2 mins stars level 8
2 mins SLH level 7	2 mins stars level 7	2 mins SLH level 7	1 min SLH level 9
1 min stars level 9	1 min SLH level 9	1 min stars level 9	2 mins stars level 7
2 mins SLH level 8	2 mins stars level 8	2 mins SLH level 8	1 min SLH level 9
–	–	1 min stars level 9	2 mins stars level 7

your speed to the intensity required. [s]oftly and move your arms as if running.

[h]igh knees Bring your knees up level with [hip]s with each step.

SU = step up Step onto a step or box with one leg at a time, then step down one leg at a time
SB = shadow boxing run on the spot but punch forwards with one arm, then the other. Hold weights or water bottles to raise the difficultly.

Beginner repeat twice a week

Week 1	Week 2	Week 3	Week 4
1 min level 5	1 min level 6	1 min SU level 6	1 min SB level 6
1 min SU level 6	1 min SB level 7	1 min SB level 8	1 min HK level 9
1 min level 6	1 min SU level 8	1 min level 6	1 min level 6
1 min SB level 8	1 min level 5	1 min HK level 8	1 min SU level 8
1 min HK level 6	1 min HK level 7	1 min level 6	1 min level 6
1 min level 8	1 min level 8	1 min SB level 8	1 min HK level 9
1 min level 6	1 min level 5	1 min level 6	1 min level 6
1 min SU level 7	1 min SB level 7	1 min HK level 9	1 min SU level 8
1 min level 9	1 min SU level 9	1 min level 6	1 min level 6
1 min HK level 6	1 min level 7	1 min SU level 9	1 min level 9

Beginner repeat twice a week

Week 1	Week 2	Week 3	Week 4
2 mins level 4	2 mins level 5	2 mins level 6	2 mins level 6
1 min SU level 5	1 min SB level 7	2 mins HK level 8	2 mins SU level 6
2 mins level 6	2 mins level 6	2 mins level 6	2 mins level 6
1.5 mins SB level 8	1.5 mins HK level 8	1 min SB level 9	1 mins HK level 9
2 mins level 6	2 mins level 6	2 mins level 6	2 mins level 7
1.5 mins HK level 8	1.5 mins level 8	1.5 mins level 8	2 mins SB level 8
2 mins level 6	2 mins SB level 6	2 mins level 6	2 mins level 6
1.5 mins SU level 7	1.5 mins level 8	1 min SU level 9	1 min HK level 9
1 min level 9	1 min HK level 9	2 mins level 6	2 mins level 7
2 mins level 6	2 mins level 7	1 min HK level 9	1 min level 9
1.5 mins HK level 7	1.5 mins SU level 8	2 mins level 6	2 mins SU level 7
2 mins level 6	2 mins level 6	1.5 mins level 8	1 min level 8

Intermediate repeat three times a week

Week 1	Week 2	Week 3	Week 4
1 min level 6	1 min level 6	1 min level 6	1 min SB level 7
1 min HK level 8	1 min SB level 9	1 min SU level 8	1 min SU level 9
1 min level 6	1 min level 6	1 min SB level 9	1 min level 8
1 min SU level 8	1 min HK level 8	1 min level 6	1 min HK level 7
1 min level 6	1 min level 6	1 min HK level 8	1 min level 8
1 min SB level 8	1 min SU level 9	1 min SU level 9	1 min SB level 9
1 min level 6	1 min level 6	1 min level 6	1 min HK level 8
1 min HK level 9	1 min HK level 9	1 min level 8	1 min level 7
1 min level 6	1 min level 6	1 min HK level 7	1 min SB level 9
1 min SU level 9	1 min SB level 9	1 min level 7	1 min level 7

Intermediate repeat three times a week

Week 1	Week 2	Week 3	Week 4
2 mins SU level 6	2 mins SB level 6	2 mins HK level 6	2 mins SU level 7
1.5 mins level 8	1.5 mins level 9	1.5 mins level 8	1 min level 9
2 mins SB level 6	2 mins HK level 6	1 min SU level 9	2 mins HK level 8
1.5 mins level 8	1.5 mins level 8	2 mins level 6	2 mins level 7
2 mins SB level 6	2 mins HK level 6	1.5 mins SU level 8	1.5 mins SB level 8
2 mins HK level 6	2 mins SU level 6	2 mins SB level 6	1.5 mins HK level 8
1 min level 9	1 min level 9	1.5 mins level 8	2 mins level 7
2 mins SU level 6	2 mins HK level 6	1 min level 9	1 min SB level 9
1 min level 9	1 min level 9	2 mins level 7	2 mins level 7
2 mins level 7	2 mins level 7	1.5 mins level 8	2 mins level 8
1.5 mins SU level 8	1.5 mins SB level 8	2 mins HK level 7	1 min SU level 9
1.5 mins level 8	1.5 mins level 8	2 mins level 8	2 mins level 7

Advanced repeat four times a week

Week 1	Week 2	Week 3	Week 4
1 min level 6	1 min level 7	1 min SU level 7	1 min level 7
1 min HK level 8	1 min HK level 9	1 min level 9	1 min SU level 9
1 min SU level 9	1 min SU level 8	1 min HK level 8	1 min level 8
1 min level 6	1 min level 7	1 min level 9	1 min HK level 9
1 min SB level 8	1 min SU level 9	1 min SB level 7	1 min level 8
1 min HK level 9	1 min level 9	1 min level 9	1 min SB level 9
1 min level 6	1 min HK level 8	1 min HK level 8	1 min level 7
1 min level 8	1 min level 7	1 min level 9	1 min HK level 9
1 min SU level 9	1 min SU level 9	1 min SU level 8	1 min level 8
1 min SB level 7	1 min level 7	1 min level 7	1 min SU level 9

Advanced repeat four times a week

Week 1	Week 2	Week 3	Week 4
2 mins level 6	2 mins level 7	2 mins level 7	2 mins level 7
2 mins HK level 8	1 min HK level 9	1 min HK level 9	1 min HK level 9
1 min level 9	2 mins level 8	2 mins level 8	2 mins level 8
2 mins SU level 6	2 mins SB level 7	1 mins SU level 9	1 min SB level 9
2 mins level 8	2 mins level 8	2 mins level 7	2 mins level 8
1 min HK level 9	1 min HK level 9	1 min HK level 9	1 min HK level 9
2 mins level 6	2 mins level 8	2 mins level 8	2 mins level 7
2 mins SB level 8	2 mins SB level 7	1 min SB level 9	1 min SB level 9
1 min SU level 9	1 min SU level 9	2 mins SU level 8	2 mins SU level 8
2 mins level 7	2 mins level 7	2 mins level 7	1 min level 9
1 min HK level 9	1 min HK level 9	1 min HK level 9	2 mins HK level 7
2 mins level 8	2 mins level 8	2 mins SU level 8	1 min SU level 9

Use any dance style you like and increase the speed according to the intensity required.

You might change the tempo of the song match the changing intensity of the prog

Beginner repeat twice a week

Week 1	Week 2	Week 3	Week 4
2 mins level 7	2 mins level 8	2 mins level 8	2 mins level 8
1 min marching level 5	1 min marching level 6	1 min marching level 6	1 min level 6
2 mins level 8	3 mins level 7	3 mins level 8	3 mins level 8
1 min marching level 5	1 min marching level 5	1 min level 6	1 min level 6
2 mins level 7	2 mins level 8	2 mins level 8	2 mins level 9
1 min marching level 5	1 min level 6	1 min level 6	1 min level 7
1 min level 9	–	–	–

Beginner repeat twice a week

Week 1	Week 2	Week 3	Week 4
3 mins level 7	2 mins level 8	2 mins level 8	2 mins level 8
1 min marching level 5	1 min marching level 6	1 min marching level 6	1 min level 6
2 mins level 8	3 mins level 7	3 mins level 8	3 mins level 8
1 min marching level 5	1 min marching level 5	1 min level 6	1 min level 6
3 mins level 7	2 mins level 8	2 mins level 8	2 mins level 9
1 min marching level 5	1 min level 6	1 min level 6	1 min level 7
1 mins level 9	2 mins level 8	1 min level 9	2 mins level 8
1 min level 6	1 min level 6	1 min level 6	1 min level 6
3 mins level 7	3 mins level 7	2 mins level 8	3 mins level 8
1 min level 6	1 min level 5	1 min level 6	2 mins level 7
2 mins level 8	2 mins level 8	3 mins level 8	2 mins level 8
1 mins level 6	1 min level 6	2 mins level 7	–

Intermediate repeat three times a week

Week 1	Week 2	Week 3	Week 4
2 mins level 8	2 mins level 8	2 mins level 9	2 mins level 9
1 min level 6	1 min level 7	1 min level 6	1 min level 7
2 mins level 9	3 mins level 8	3 mins level 8	3 mins level 8
1 min level 6	1 min level 5	1 min level 6	1 min level 7
2 mins level 8	2 mins level 9	2 mins level 8	2 mins level 9
1 min level 6	1 min level 7	1 min level 6	1 min level 8
1 min level 9	–	–	–

Intermediate repeat three times a week

Week 1	Week 2	Week 3	Week 4
2 mins level 8	2 mins level 8	2 mins level 9	2 mins level 9
1 min level 6	1 min level 7	1 min level 6	1 min level 7
2 mins level 9	3 mins level 8	3 mins level 8	3 mins level 8
1 min level 6	1 min level 5	1 min level 6	1 min level 7
2 mins level 8	2 mins level 9	2 mins level 8	2 mins level 9
1 min level 6	1 min level 7	1 min level 6	1 min level 8
1 min level 9	1 min level 9	2 mins level 9	1 min level 7
3 mins level 8	2 mins level 8	1 min level 6	2 mins level 8
1 min level 7	1 min level 7	2 mins level 8	1 min level 9
1 min level 9	2 mins level 8	1 min level 7	1 min level 7
2 mins level 8	1 min level 7	1 min level 9	3 mins level 8
1 min level 6	1 min level 9	2 mins level 8	1 min level 7
2 mins level 8	2 mins level 8	1 min level 7	1 min level 9

Advanced repeat four times a week

Week 1	Week 2	Week 3	Week 4
3 mins level 8	3 mins level 8	3 mins level 9	3 mins level 9
1 min level 6	1 min level 7	1 min level 7	1 min level 7
2 mins level 9	3 mins level 8	3 mins level 8	3 mins level 9
1 min level 6	1 min level 7	1 min level 7	1 min level 6
3 mins level 8	2 mins level 9	2 mins level 9	2 mins level 9

Advanced repeat four times a week

Week 1	Week 2	Week 3	Week 4
3 mins level 8	3 mins level 8	3 mins level 9	3 mins level 9
1 min level 6	1 min level 7	1 min level 7	1 min level 7
2 mins level 9	3 mins level 8	3 mins level 8	3 mins level 9
1 min level 6	1 min level 7	1 min level 7	1 min level 6
3 mins level 8	2 mins level 9	2 mins level 9	2 mins level 9
2 mins level 7	2 mins level 7	1 min level 7	1 min level 7
1 min level 9	3 mins level 8	2 mins level 9	2 mins level 9
1 min level 6	1 min level 7	1 min level 7	1 min level 8
2 mins level 8	2 mins level 8	2 mins level 8	1 min level 9
2 mins level 7	1 min level 7	2 mins level 7	2 mins level 7
2 mins level 8	1 min level 9	2 mins level 9	3 mins level 8

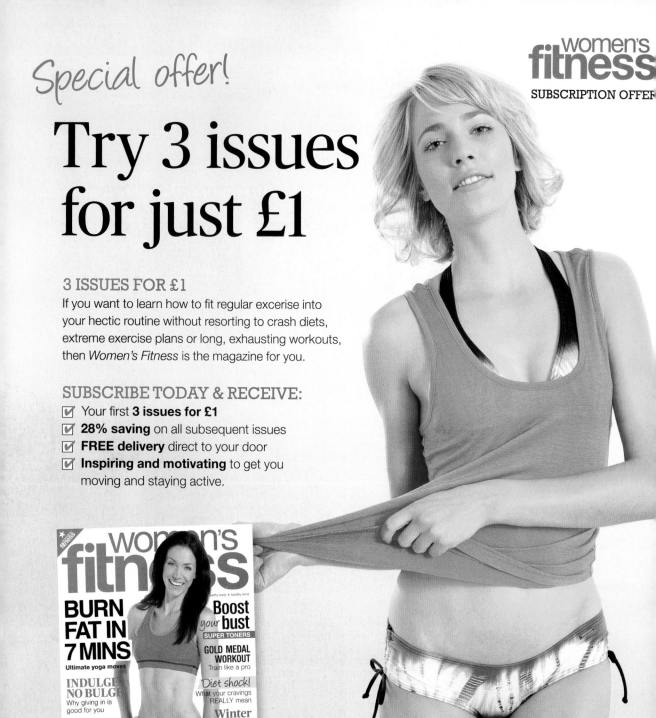

Tone your tum

Our top 10 exercises target every inch of your tummy. Washboard abs, here you come!

Stomach

stomach v-sit

Areas trained: Stomach, core

Technique

- Sit on the floor with knees bent and your arms by your sides.
- Lift both feet off the floor and bend your knees to 90 degrees. This is the start position.
- Straighten your legs and lower your body to create a 'v' shape. Hold for a count of five.
- Lift up to the start position and repeat.

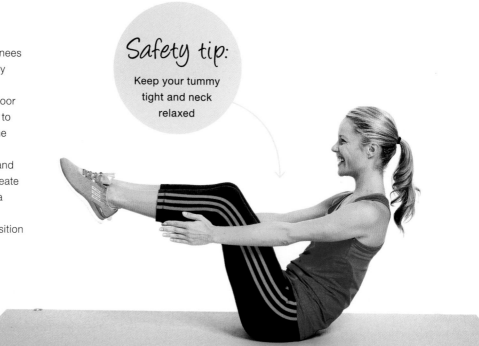

Safety tip: Keep your tummy tight and neck relaxed

44

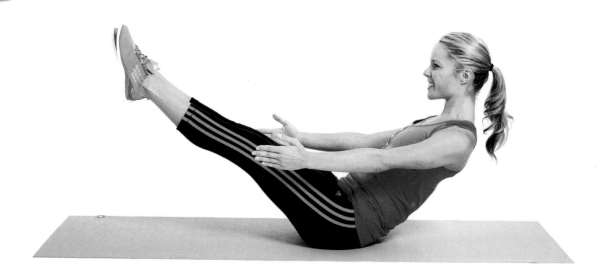

Areas trained: Stomach, core, bottom

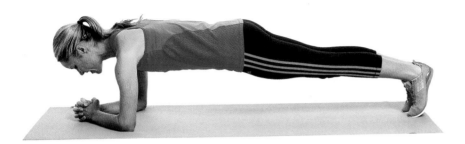

Technique

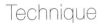

- Lie on your stomach with your elbows directly underneath your shoulders.
- Lift your body off the floor onto your elbows and toes into the plank position.
- Bend your left knee and lift your foot to the sky while holding the plank position.
- Beginners repeat for 15 seconds on the left side, then 15 seconds on the right; intermediates repeat for 20 seconds on each side; advanced for 25 seconds on each side.

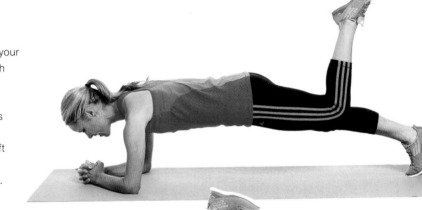

45

Safety tip:

Keep your tummy tight and don't allow your lower back to sag

Area trained: Stomach

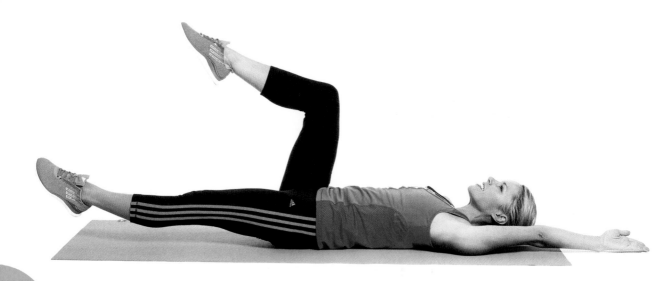

Technique

46

- Lie on your back with your right knee lifted and bent to a 90-degree angle and your left leg straight.
- Extend your left arm behind your head and either support your head with your right hand or leave it on the floor.
- Crunch your body up, so that your left arm reaches towards your left ankle.
- Lower down with control.
- Beginners repeat for 15 seconds on the left side, then 15 seconds on the right; intermediates repeat for 20 seconds on each side; advanced for 25 seconds on each side.

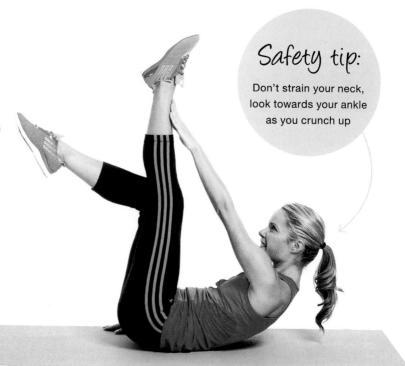

Safety tip:

Don't strain your neck, look towards your ankle as you crunch up

Areas trained: Core muscles, back

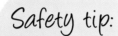

Safety tip:

Keep your tummy tight
and your arm and leg at
an even height

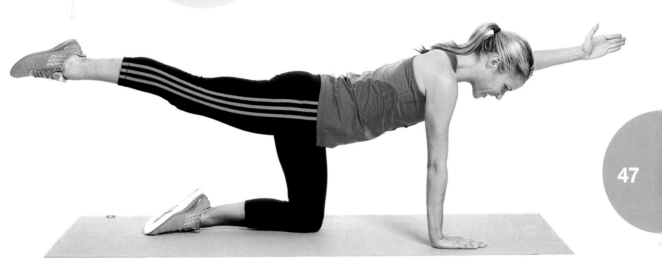

47

Technique

- Kneel on all fours.
- Extend your left arm out in front of you
  and your right leg out behind you and
  hold for a count of two, keeping your back
  and hips level.
- Lower your leg and arm and repeat on the
  other side. Continue, alternating sides.

stomach toe touch

Area trained: Stomach

Technique

- Begin lying on your back with arms extended by your sides, feet lifted off the floor and hips and knees bent to 90 degrees.
- Lift your head, shoulders and arms off the floor, crunching your stomach in and bringing your upper body off the floor towards your thighs.
- Holding this position, lower your left toe towards the floor, then back up, then repeat on the other side. Continue, alternating sides.

48

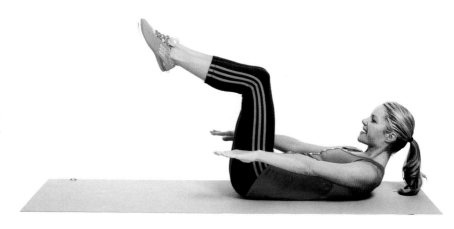

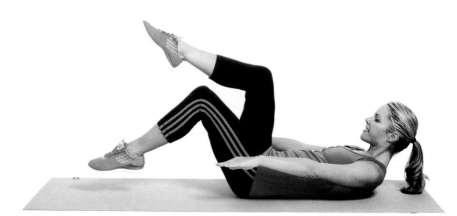

Safety tip:

Keep your neck relaxed and don't allow your chin to come towards your chest

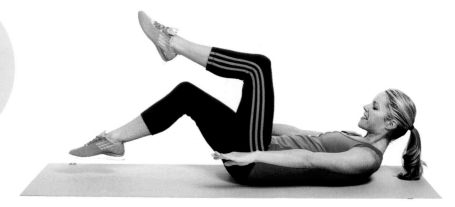

Areas trained: Stomach, side muscles

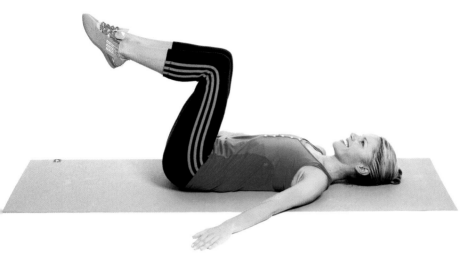

Technique

- Lie on your back with your arms spread, feet lifted, and hips and knees bent to 90 degrees.
- Gently lower both legs down to the left until they are just above the floor.
- Bring them back to centre, over to the right and finally back to centre. Repeat.

49

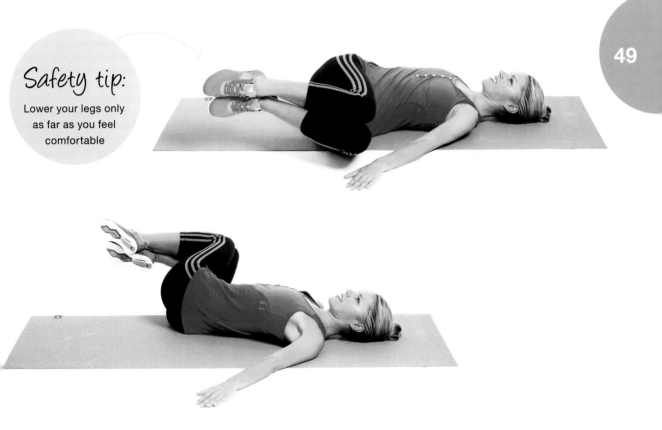

Safety tip:
Lower your legs only as far as you feel comfortable

Area trained: Stomach

Technique

- Begin in a plank position, body lifted on your hands and toes with your arms straight, keeping a straight line from shoulders to feet.
- Keeping your stomach pulled in, lift your left foot and bring your left knee towards your right elbow.
- Slowly straighten the leg, return your foot to the start position and repeat the movement with your right leg. Keep alternating legs.
- Make sure you keep your shoulders level throughout each movement.

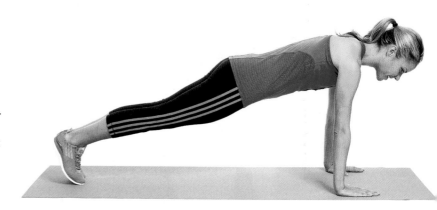

50

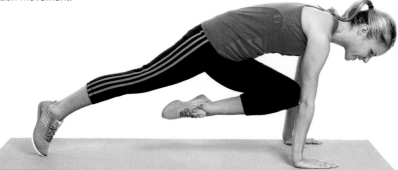

Safety tip:

Don't allow your hips to sag and keep your shoulders directly above your hands

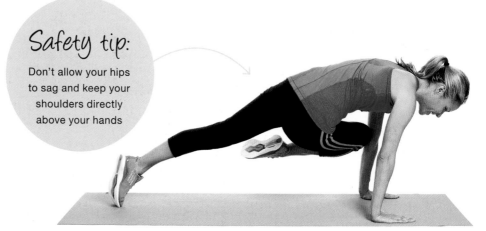

Area trained: Stomach

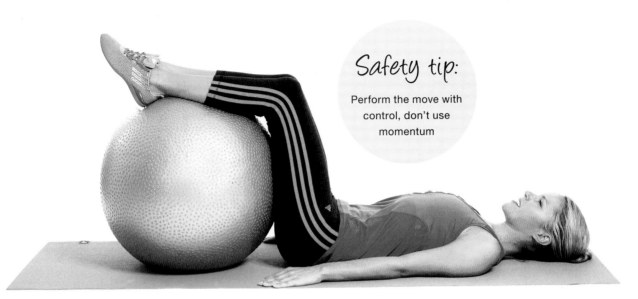

Safety tip:

Perform the move with control, don't use momentum

51

Technique

- Lie on your back with your arms by your sides and rest your lower legs on a stability ball, knees bent.
- Tuck your heels into the ball and push it against your thighs.
- Tighten your stomach muscles and lift the ball off the floor with your legs, bringing it towards your body.
- Lower, but don't let the ball rest on the floor. Repeat.

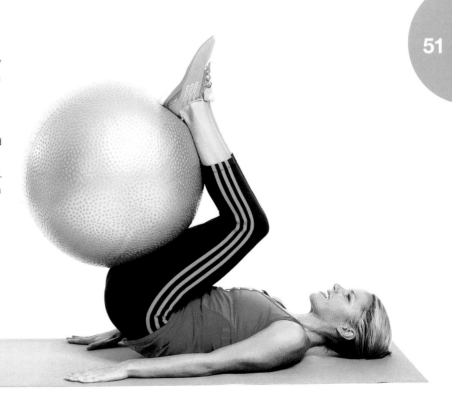

Areas trained: Stomach, side muscles, back

Technique

- Lie on your back with your hands behind your ears and extend your legs up to the ceiling.
- Crunch your shoulders up and reach your right hand towards your left foot. Lower with control.
- Crunch up again, reaching your left hand towards your right foot.
- Continue, alternating between right and left.

52

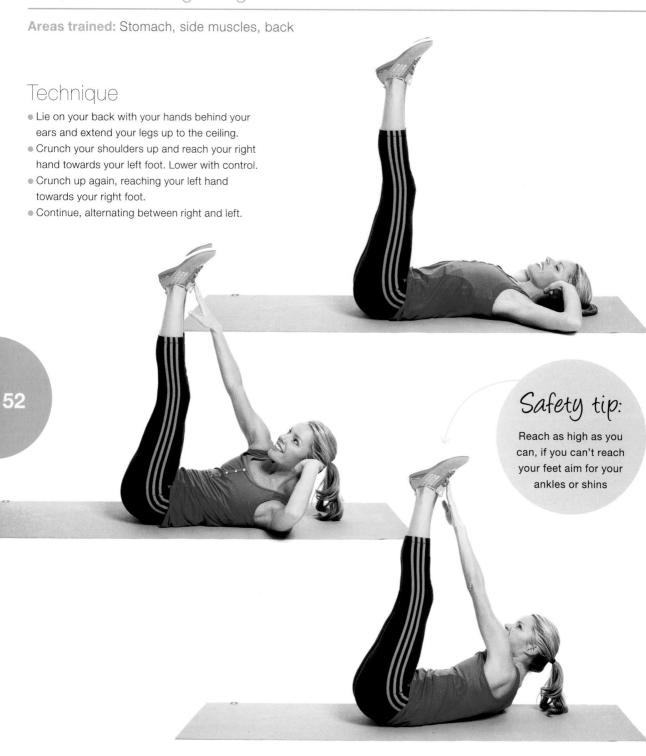

Safety tip:

Reach as high as you can, if you can't reach your feet aim for your ankles or shins

Areas trained: Stomach, core, inner thighs

Technique

- Lie on your back with your knees bent, your feet flat on the floor and your hands behind your ears.
- Place a towel between your knees. This is the start position.
- Squeeze your knees tightly together while crunching your shoulders off the floor.
- Hold the top position before slowly returning to the start position and repeating.

Safety tip:

Keep your neck relaxed and don't allow your chin to come towards your chest

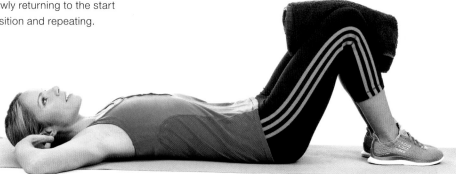

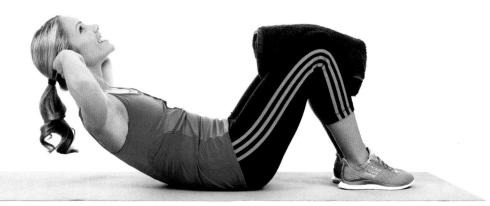

53

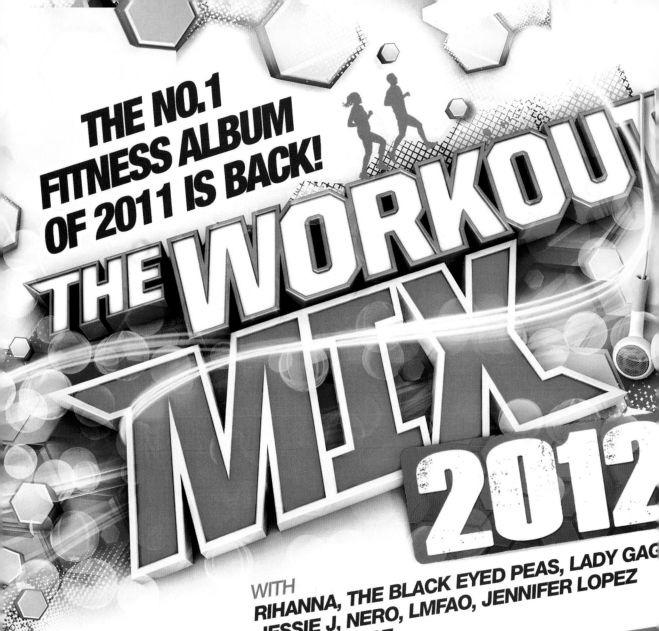

THE NO.1 FITNESS ALBUM OF 2011 IS BACK!

THE WORKOUT MIX 2012

WITH
RIHANNA, THE BLACK EYED PEAS, LADY GAG[A]
JESSIE J, NERO, LMFAO, JENNIFER LOPEZ
& MANY MORE

MIXES CREATED BY
FITNESS EXPERTS
FOR MAXIMUM RESULT[S]

FOLLOW US ON
WWW.THEWORKOUTMIX.COM
@THEWORKOUTMIX & FACEBOOK/THEWORKOUTMIX
AVAILABLE TO PRE-ORDER amazon.co.uk
OUT 26TH DECEMBER

Boost your bum

Get a gorgeously pert behind with these 10 easy moves. Your favourite jeans never looked so good!

Bottom

bottom single-leg bridge

Area trained: Bottom

Technique

- Lie on your back with your knees bent and your arms by your sides.
- Lift your left foot and straighten your leg, keeping your knees together.
- Lift your bottom off the floor. Make sure that your hips stay level.
- Hold the top position for a count of one. Lower, but don't rest your bottom on the floor, then repeat.
- Beginners repeat for 15 seconds on the right leg, then 15 seconds on the left; intermediates repeat for 20 seconds on each side; advanced for 25 seconds each side.

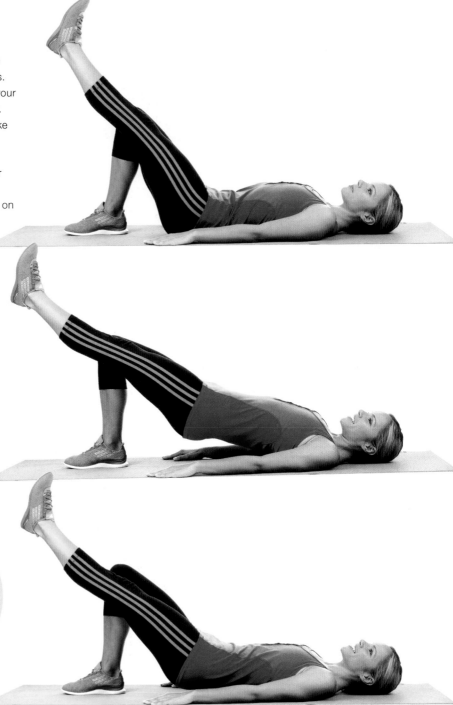

Safety tip:

Keep your tummy tight and your hips as level as possible, without dropping them

Areas trained: Bottom, back of thighs

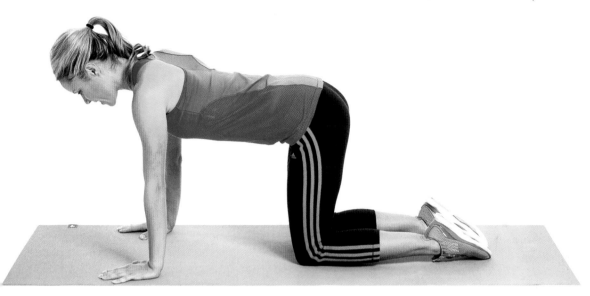

Safety tip:

Keep your tummy tight
and don't let your
lower back sag

57

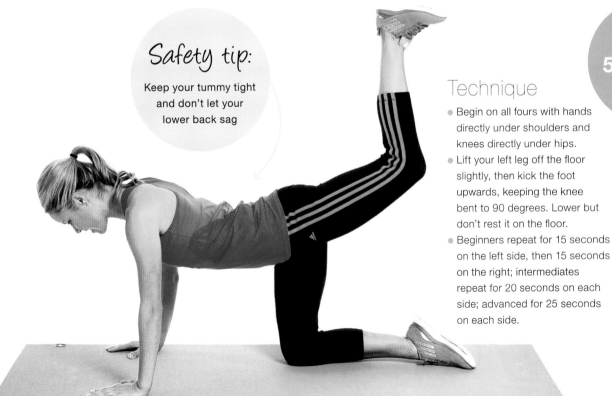

Technique

- Begin on all fours with hands directly under shoulders and knees directly under hips.
- Lift your left leg off the floor slightly, then kick the foot upwards, keeping the knee bent to 90 degrees. Lower but don't rest it on the floor.
- Beginners repeat for 15 seconds on the left side, then 15 seconds on the right; intermediates repeat for 20 seconds on each side; advanced for 25 seconds on each side.

bottom kneeling abduction

Areas trained: Bottom, outer thighs

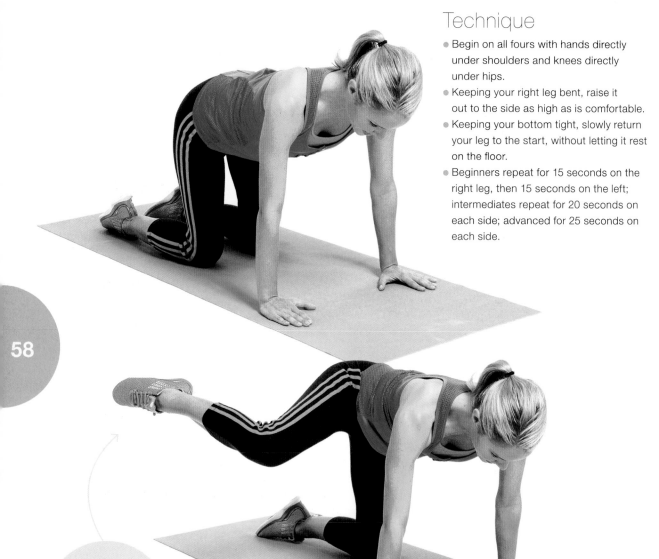

Technique

- Begin on all fours with hands directly under shoulders and knees directly under hips.
- Keeping your right leg bent, raise it out to the side as high as is comfortable.
- Keeping your bottom tight, slowly return your leg to the start, without letting it rest on the floor.
- Beginners repeat for 15 seconds on the right leg, then 15 seconds on the left; intermediates repeat for 20 seconds on each side; advanced for 25 seconds on each side.

58

Safety tip:
Only lift your leg as high as is comfortable

Areas trained: Bottom, outer thighs

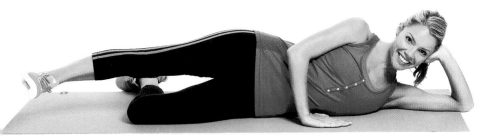

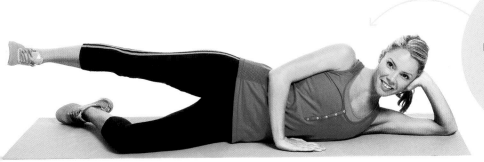

Safety tip:

Keep your hips as level as possible, without excessively rotating them as you lift your leg

59

Technique

- Lie on your left side with your left knee bent to 90 degrees and your upper body resting on your left elbow and right hand.
- Lift your right leg over left, keeping it straight and flexing the foot. This is your starting position.

- Lift your right leg up towards the ceiling, keeping your foot flexed. Lower with control.
- Beginners repeat for 15 seconds on the right leg, then 15 seconds on the left; intermediates repeat for 20 seconds on each side; advanced for 25 seconds on each side.

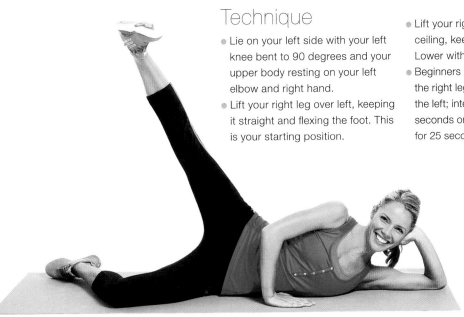

bottom pretzel

Areas trained: Bottom, outer thighs

Technique

- Lie on your left side with your knees bent to 90 degrees, your upper body propped up on your left forearm.
- Place a 2-4kg medicine ball behind your right knee and bring your right hand to the ground.
- Lift your right leg as high as you can, squeezing your lower leg towards your bum to keep the ball in place.
- Slowly lower to just above the floor. Beginners repeat for 15 seconds on the right leg, then 15 seconds on the left; intermediates repeat for 20 seconds on each side; advanced for 25 seconds on each side.

60

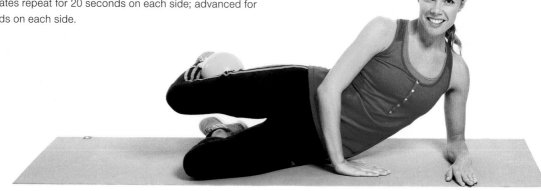

Safety tip:
Keep your upper body still at all times.

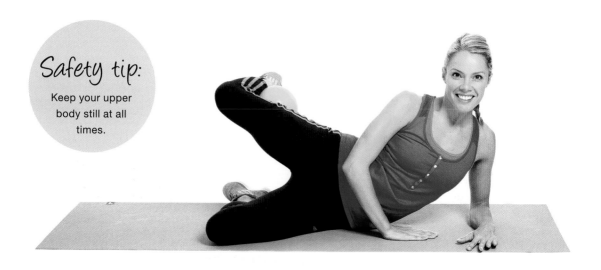

Areas trained: Bottom, lower stomach

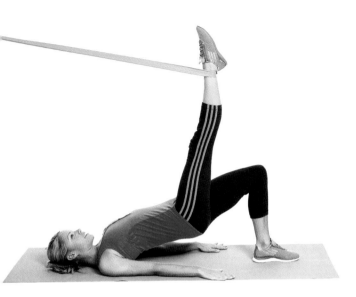

Technique

- Attach one end of a resistance band to a sturdy object around three feet from the floor. Attach the other end around your right leg, just above the ankle.
- Lie on your back with the top of your head pointing towards the resistance band then bend your knees and lift your hips. This is your starting position.
- Straighten your right leg towards the ceiling, then circle it out to the side and back up to the start, then reverse the move. Beginners repeat for 15 seconds on the right leg, then 15 seconds on the left; intermediates repeat for 20 seconds on each side; advanced for 25 seconds on each side.

61

Safety tip:

Don't allow your back to arch and keep your hips level when taking your leg to the side

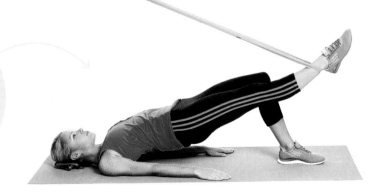

Areas trained: Bottom, inner thighs, core

Technique

- Begin lying on your back with your hips and knees bent and a medicine ball gripped between your thighs.
- Tighten your bottom slightly, raising your hips off the floor to form a straight line from shoulders to knees, while simultaneously squeezing your thighs together into the ball.
- Hold for a count of five, lower and repeat.

62

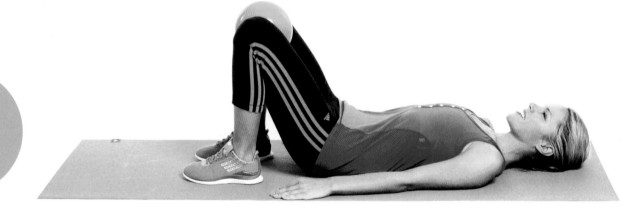

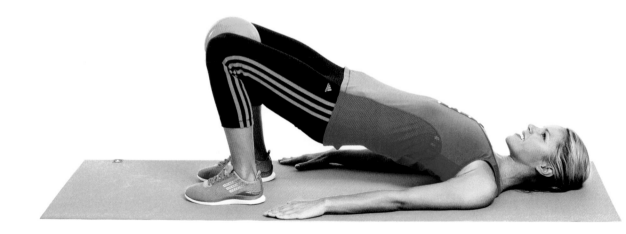

Areas trained: Bottom, thighs, core

Technique

- Begin standing with feet hip-width apart and arms straight out in front of you. Come into a half-squat position, so your hips are higher than your knees.
- Transfer your weight onto your right leg then hinge forwards from the hips (you may straighten your right knee slightly), taking your left leg straight behind you and your torso forwards.
- Hinge back to return to the half-squat position and repeat. Beginners repeat for 15 seconds on the right leg, then 15 seconds on the left; intermediates repeat for 20 seconds on each side; advanced for 25 seconds on each side.

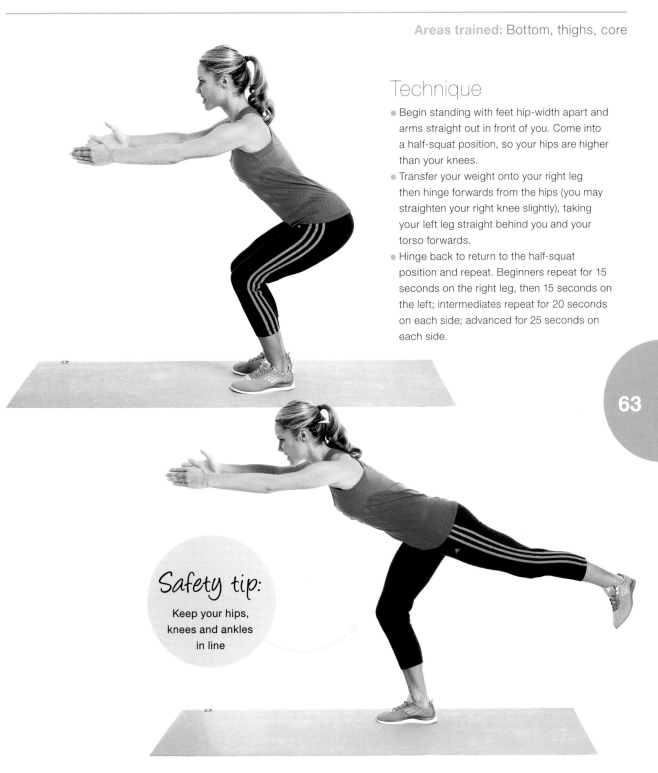

63

Safety tip:

Keep your hips, knees and ankles in line

bottom half moon

Area trained: Bottom

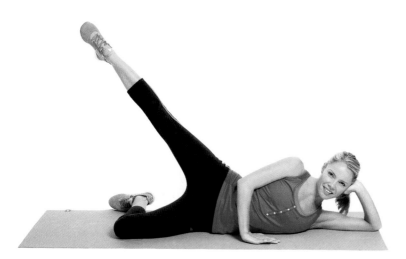

Technique

- Begin lying on your left side with your head supported by your left hand, legs extended.
- Lift your right leg so it points diagonally upwards and bend your left leg to 90 degrees – this is your start position.
- Bring your right leg down and forwards, then back to the start, then down and backwards and finally back to the start. Your leg should move in a smooth, arcing motion throughout.
- Beginners repeat for 15 seconds on the right leg, then 15 seconds on the left; intermediates repeat for 20 seconds on each side; advanced for 25 seconds on each side.

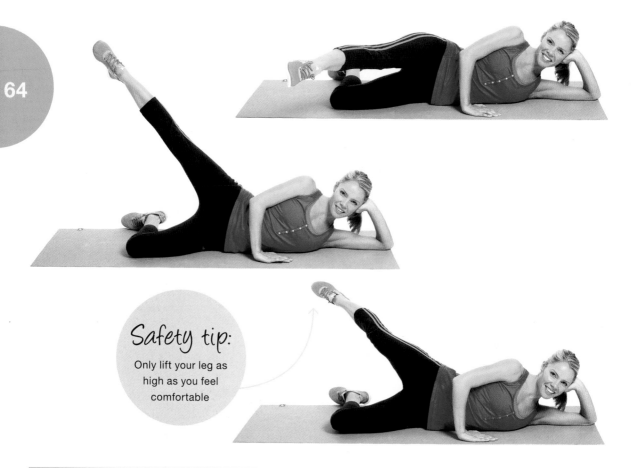

Safety tip:
Only lift your leg as high as you feel comfortable

Technique

- Begin with your upper back and head resting on a stability ball, knees bent at 90 degrees with body parallel to the floor.
- Slowly drop your bum towards the floor, bending your hips and knees. Slowly return to the start and repeat.

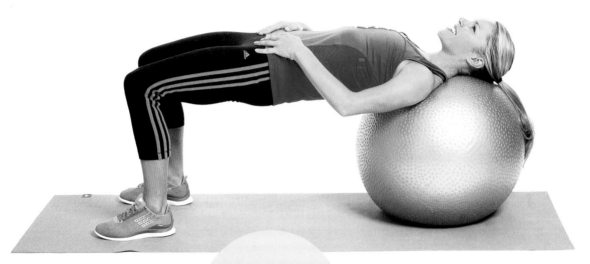

Safety tip:

Make sure your head and neck are supported throughout

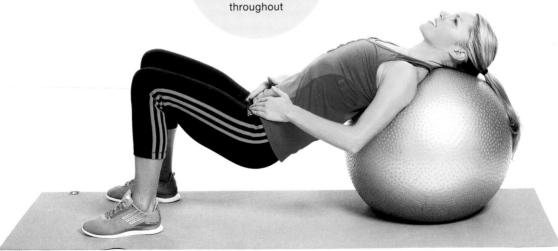

65

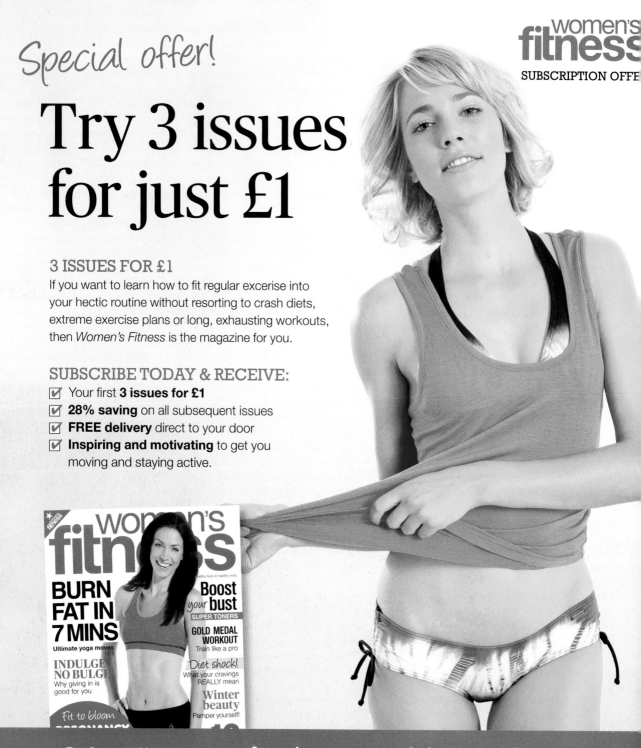

Special offer!

Try 3 issues for just £1

women's fitness
SUBSCRIPTION OFFE

3 ISSUES FOR £1

If you want to learn how to fit regular excerise into your hectic routine without resorting to crash diets, extreme exercise plans or long, exhausting workouts, then *Women's Fitness* is the magazine for you.

SUBSCRIBE TODAY & RECEIVE:

- ☑ Your first **3 issues for £1**
- ☑ **28% saving** on all subsequent issues
- ☑ **FREE delivery** direct to your door
- ☑ **Inspiring and motivating** to get you moving and staying active.

Order online at **www.dennismags.co.uk/womensfitness** or

CALL 0844 844 0246

using offer code: G1111HW

Whittle your waist

Working your waist will really define your curves, or help create them!

Waist

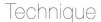

waist side knee to top elbow

Area trained: Side muscles

Technique

- Lie on your left side with your legs slightly in the air, your hands behind your head.
- Roll slightly backwards onto the soft part of your bottom.
- Tuck in your knees, bringing your right knee towards your right elbow.
- Straighten your legs, lifting your ankles towards the ceiling.
- Beginners repeat for 15 seconds on the left side, then 15 seconds on the right; intermediates repeat for 20 seconds on each side; advanced for 25 seconds on each side.

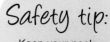

Safety tip:
Keep your neck relaxed at all times

68

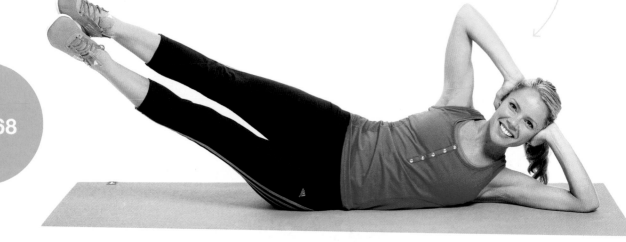

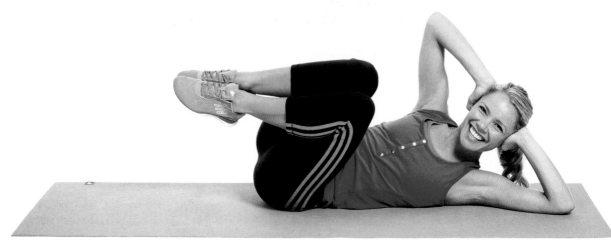

Areas trained: Side muscles, inner thighs

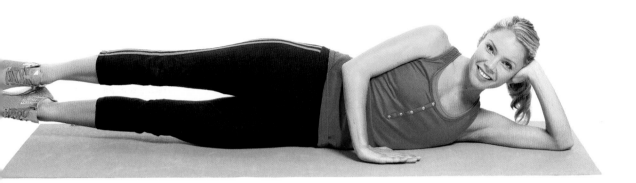

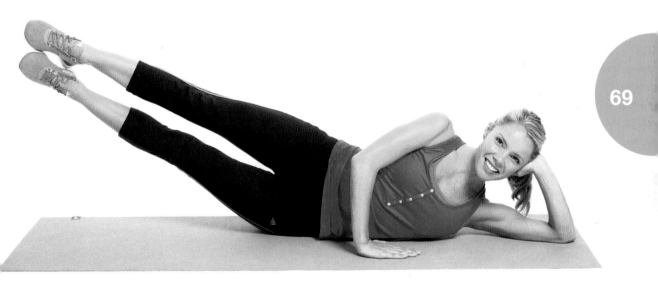

69

Safety tip:

Keep your tummy tight
and don't lift your
legs higher than is
comfortable

Technique

● Lie on your left side and place your
right hand on the floor in front of
your stomach for balance.

● Keep your feet together and lift
your legs off the floor as high as
you can.

● Keep your legs straight and hold

the top position for a count of one.

● Lower your legs to touch the floor
but don't rest them, then repeat.
Beginners repeat for 15 seconds on
the left side, then 15 seconds on
the right; intermediates repeat for
20 seconds on each side; advanced
for 25 seconds on each side.

Areas trained: Side muscles, stomach

Technique

- Start lying on your left side, legs in line with your hips and shoulders, with feet together.
- Place your left forearm on the floor, directly under your shoulder.
- Lift your hips off the floor to form a straight line from head to toe, taking your right arm up into the air.
- Beginners repeat for 15 seconds on the left side, then 15 seconds on the right; intermediates repeat for 20 seconds on each side; advanced for 25 seconds on each side.

Safety tip:

Keep your body in a straight line and don't allow your hips to sag

70

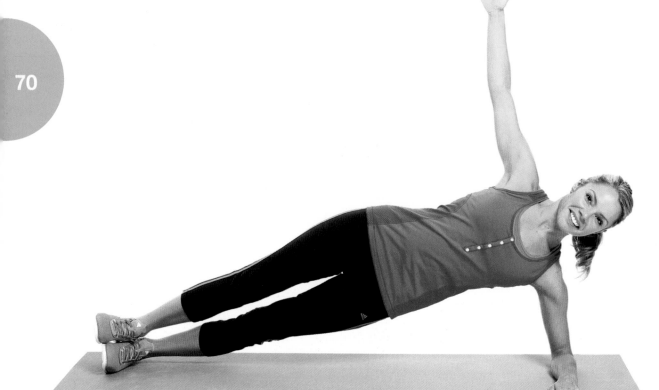

Areas trained: Side muscles, stomach

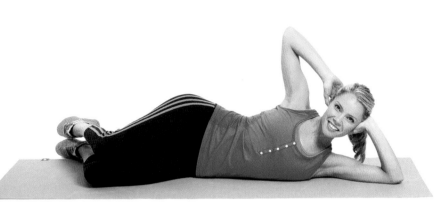

Technique

- Lie on your left side, and lift your upper body slightly, bringing your hands to your ears. Bend your knees inwards, until your heels are in line with your bottom. This is your start position.
- Crunch your right knee towards your right elbow, then extend the right leg.
- Beginners repeat for 15 seconds on the left side, then 15 seconds on the right; intermediates repeat for 20 seconds on each side; advanced for 25 seconds on each side.

71

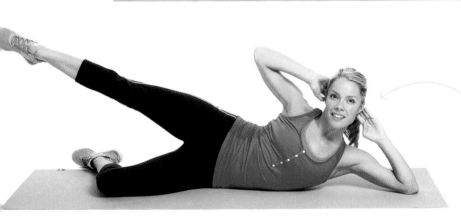

Safety tip:

Keep your neck relaxed and your lifted ankle in line with your hips

waist side bends

Area trained: Side muscles

Technique

- Stand with your feet shoulder-width apart holding a dumbbell in each hand, lifted above your head.
- Tighten your stomach and lean over to your right, as far as you feel comfortable.
- Come back to the centre, then over to the left. Continue, alternating sides.

Safety tip:

Make sure you don't lean forward or back during the movement

72

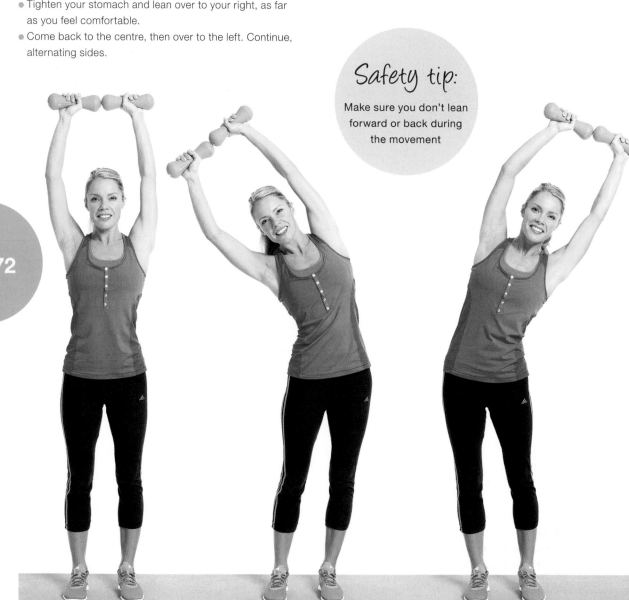

Areas trained: Side muscles, lower stomach

Technique

- Begin by sitting on the floor with your knees bent and your feet flat on the floor. Extend your arms out in front of you, shoulder-width apart.
- Lean back so your body is at about a 45-degree angle to the floor.
- Keeping your lower body still, twist your upper body to the right, then to the left. Continue, alternating sides.

73

Safety tip:

The more you lean back, the harder the exercise becomes, so choose an angle that's comfortable but still challenges your muscles

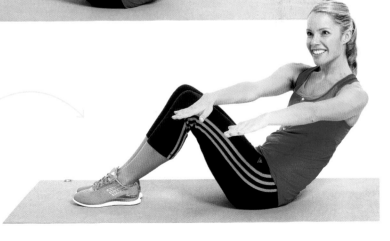

waist bicycle

Technique

- Lie flat on the floor with your lower back pressed to the ground, hands resting by your sides. Lift your legs and bend your knees to 90 degrees.
- Slowly bend your left knee towards your chest and bring your right elbow to meet it
- Straighten your left leg, and bring your right knee towards your left elbow simultaneously.
- Continue alternating sides in a cycling motion.

Safety tip:

Keep your neck long and don't pull on your head, rest your hands by your ears

74

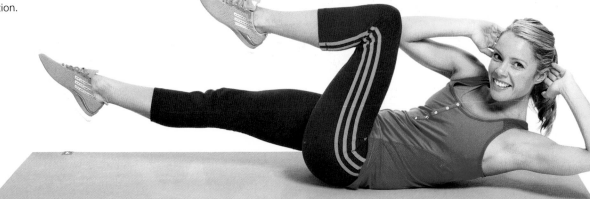

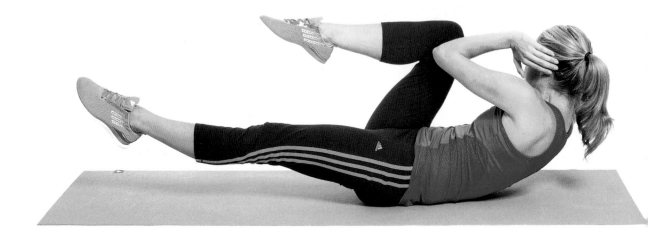

Areas trained: Side muscles, stomach

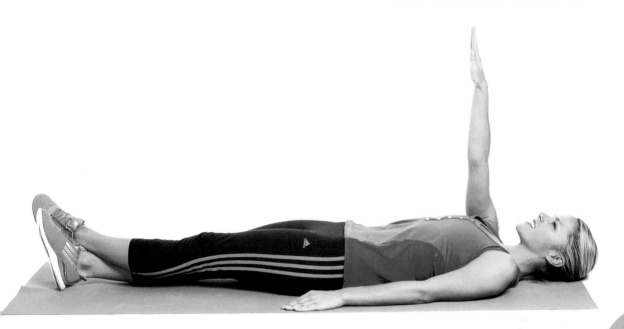

75

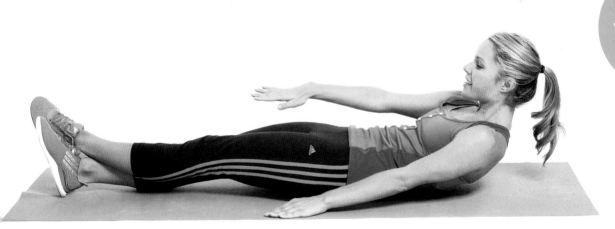

Technique

- Begin lying on your back with straight legs, left ankle crossed over your right.
- Lift your right arm up, then tighten your stomach muscles and reach it up and across the centre of your body.
- Hold for a count of one then lower down. Change the cross of your legs, lift the left arm and repeat. Continue, alternating.

Safety tip:

Keep your lower back pressed into the floor

waist woodchopper

Area trained: Side muscles

Technique

- Begin standing with feet shoulder-width apart, holding a medicine ball overhead with both hands.
- Quickly bring the ball down and across your body towards your right ankle, bending your hips and knees as you do so.
- Bring the ball up to return to the start then repeat the move to the left side. Continue, alternating sides.

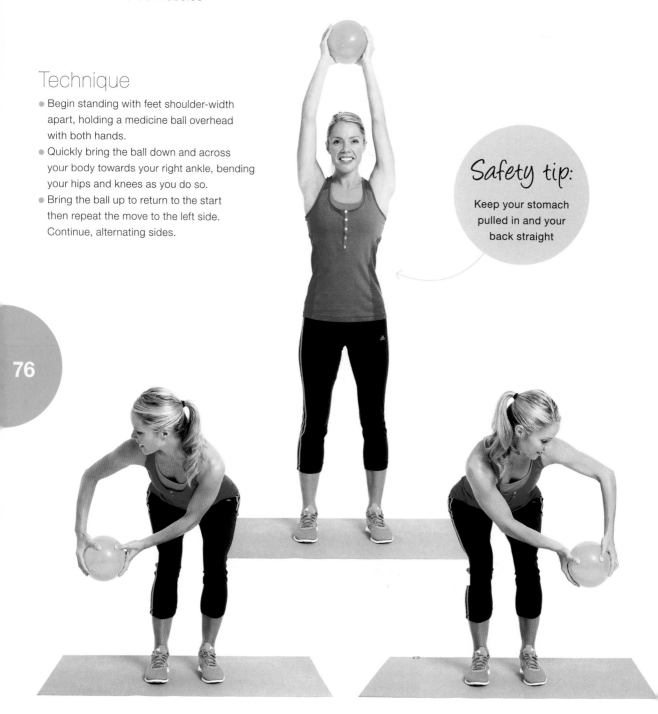

Safety tip:

Keep your stomach pulled in and your back straight

Areas trained: Side muscles, core, balance

Technique

- Lie in a straight line on your left side.
- Place your left elbow beneath your left shoulder and extend your right arm to the ceiling.
- Lift your hips off the floor into the side plank position.
- Slowly lower your right arm and thread it between your left arm and the floor.
- Return to the start position. Beginners repeat for 15 seconds on the left side, then 15 seconds on the right; intermediates repeat for 20 seconds on each side; advanced for 25 seconds on each side.

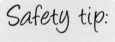

Safety tip:
Keep your tummy tight and don't allow your hips to sag

77

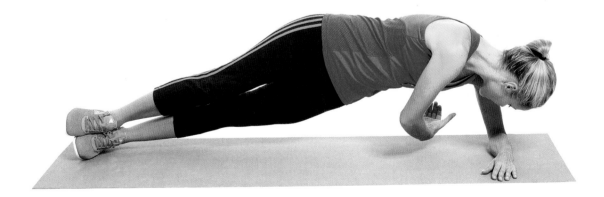

Slim your pins!

Sculpt, shape and strengthen your legs with these hip-to-toe toners

Legs

Area trained: Back of upper thighs

Technique

- Lie on your back with your lower legs on a stability ball, arms by your sides.
- Tighten your stomach and bottom to raise your hips, making a straight line with your shoulders, hips and toes. This is the start position.
- Bring your heels towards your bottom, pointing your toes away from you so the soles of your feet rest on the ball.
- Continue to pull your heels towards you, raising your hips further off the floor, then lower slowly back to the start position and repeat.

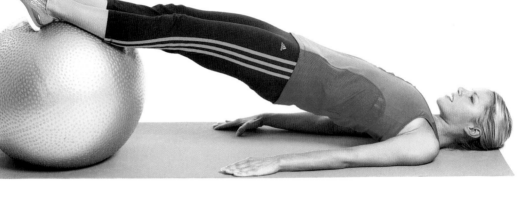

79

Safety tip:

Keep your neck relaxed and your head still

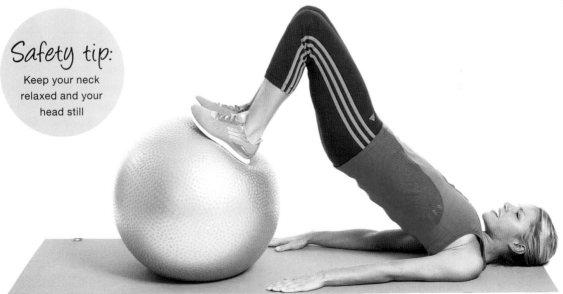

legs standing calf raises

Areas trained: Calves, front of thighs

Technique

- Stand with your heels off the floor, resting your weight on the balls of your feet.
- Keeping your chest raised, slowly squat downwards, lifting your heels further upwards and bringing your weight forward onto your toes. Hold for a count of five.
- Carefully lower your heels to the floor, then lift up back to the start position. Repeat.
- To make the exercise harder, hold a dumbbell in each hand.

Safety tip:

Keep your back straight and your stomach muscles tight

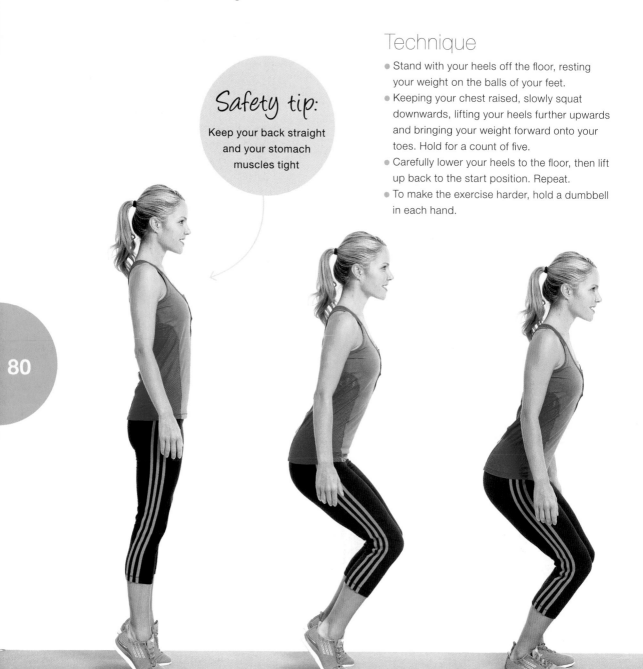

80

Areas trained: Front and outer thighs, bottom

Technique

- Stand with your feet together, holding a pair of dumbbells by your thighs. This is the start position.
- Squat down, bending your hips and knees at the same time, as if you were going to sit on an imaginary chair.
- Push through your heels, straighten your legs and return to the start position. Keep looking straight ahead and repeat.

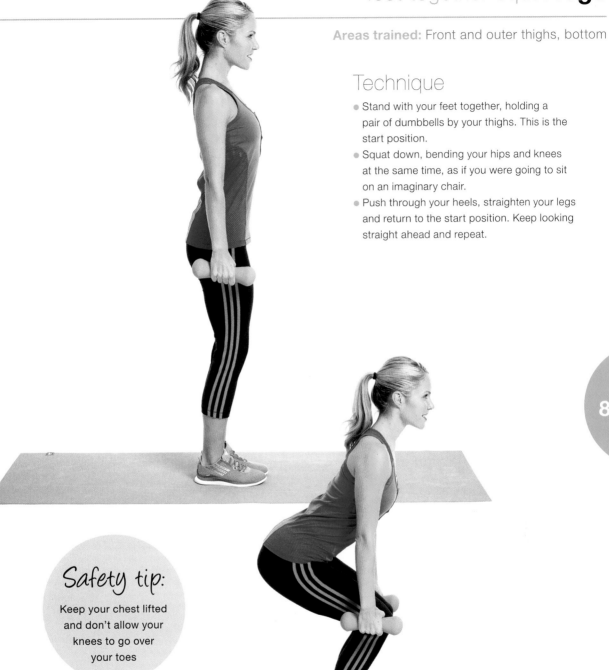

81

Safety tip:

Keep your chest lifted and don't allow your knees to go over your toes

Area trained: Front of shins

Technique

- Tie the ends of a resistance band together to form a circle. Secure one end around a sturdy object such as a table leg, just above the floor.
- Sit on the floor facing the table, with your right leg extended and the band around the top of your right foot. There should be a little tension in the band.

This is your start position.
- Draw your right toes up as far as you can towards your shin, then return to the start position
- Beginners repeat for 15 seconds on the right side, then 15 seconds on the left; intermediates repeat for 20 seconds on each side; advanced repeat for 25 seconds on each side.

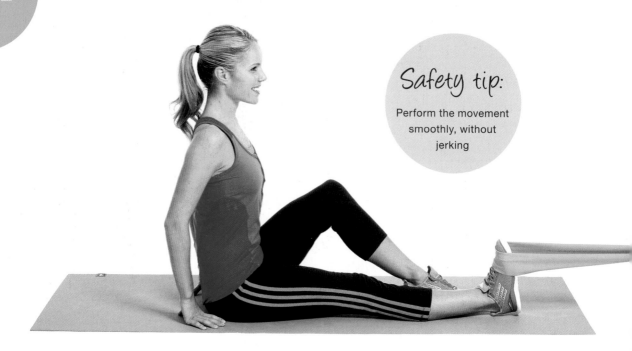

Safety tip:

Perform the movement smoothly, without jerking

Areas trained: Front of thighs, bottom, cardio fitness

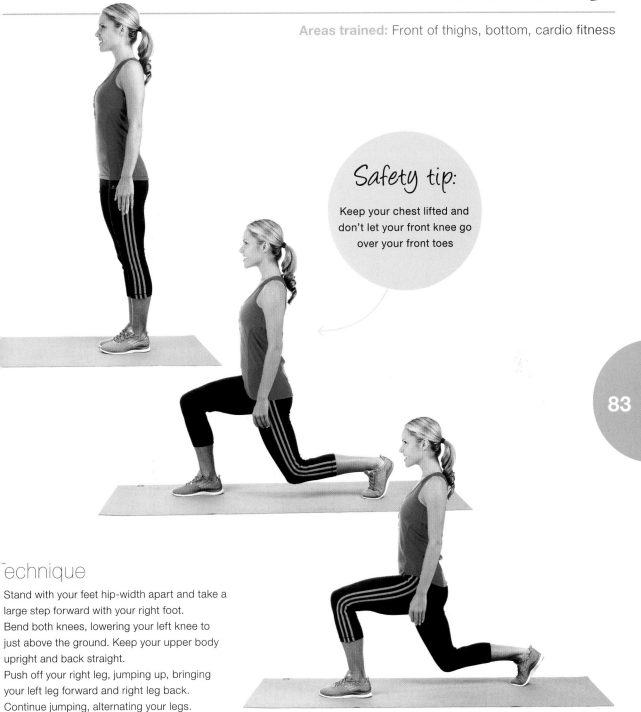

Safety tip:

Keep your chest lifted and don't let your front knee go over your front toes

83

Technique

Stand with your feet hip-width apart and take a large step forward with your right foot.
Bend both knees, lowering your left knee to just above the ground. Keep your upper body upright and back straight.
Push off your right leg, jumping up, bringing your left leg forward and right leg back.
Continue jumping, alternating your legs.

Areas trained: Thighs, bottom

Technique

- Begin standing with your feet hip-width apart, arms extended in front of you.
- Lift your left foot off the floor in front of you and transfer your weight to your right leg.
- Bend your right hip and knee, sitting back and squatting down. Extend your left leg so that the thigh is at a 45-degree angle to the floor.
- Push through your right heel and return to the start.
- Beginners repeat for 15 seconds on the right side, then 15 seconds on the left; intermediates repeat for 20 seconds on each side; advanced repeat for 25 seconds on each side.

84

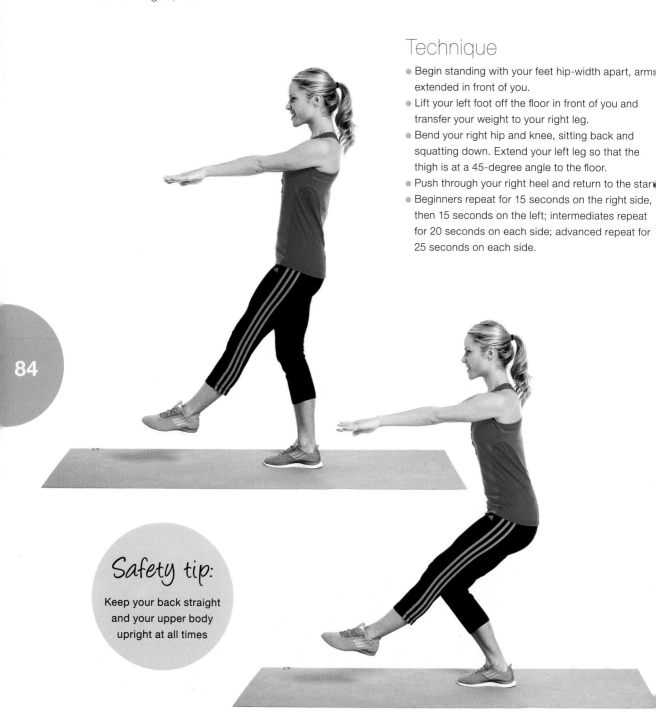

Safety tip:

Keep your back straight and your upper body upright at all times

Technique

- Lie on your left side with your left knee bent to 90 degrees and your right leg lifted and extended straight out.
- Moving clockwise, draw a figure-of-eight shape with your right leg four times.
- Repeat four times anticlockwise, then change legs. Beginners repeat for 15 seconds on the right side, then 15 seconds on the left; intermediates repeat for 20 seconds on each side; advanced repeat for 25 seconds on each side.

Safety tip:

Keep your hips square and in line with your shoulders at all times

85

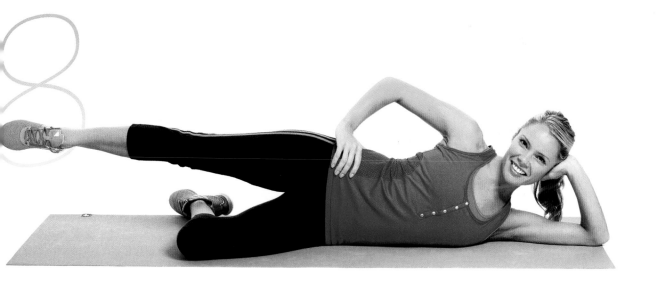

legs resistance band leg press

Areas trained: Legs, lower stomach

Technique

- Begin lying on your back with a resistance band looped around your feet, holding an end in each hand. Bring your knees in towards your chest with your arms by your sides.
- Straighten your legs out to around a 45-degree angle to the floor, then slowly return to the start and repeat.

Safety tip:

Keep your lower back pressed into the floor throughout

86

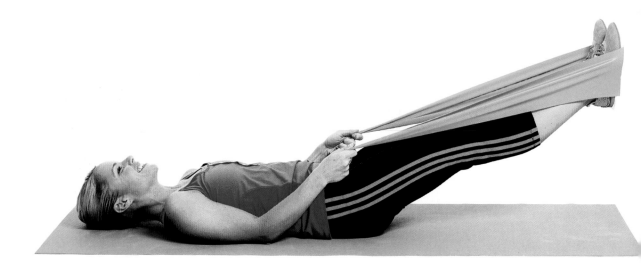

Areas trained: Bottom, front of thighs

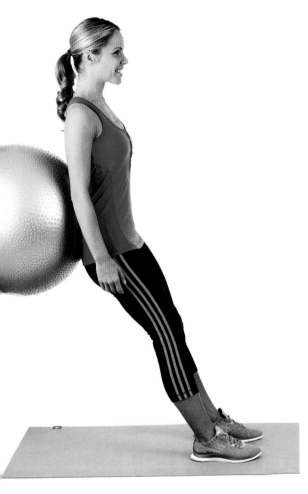

Technique

- Place a stability ball against a wall and stand resting against it, facing away from the wall so that your lower back is supported by the ball. Keep your feet shoulder-width apart and slightly in front of your shoulders.
- Squat down so your hips and knees are bent to 90 degrees, then stand halfway up and repeat.

87

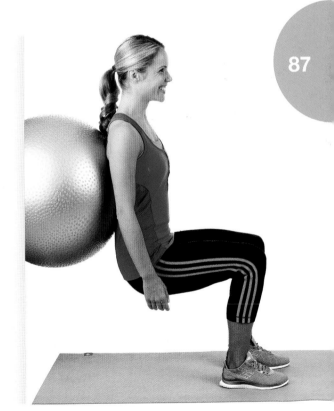

Safety tip:

Keep your chest lifted and your knees and ankles aligned

Area trained: Inner thighs

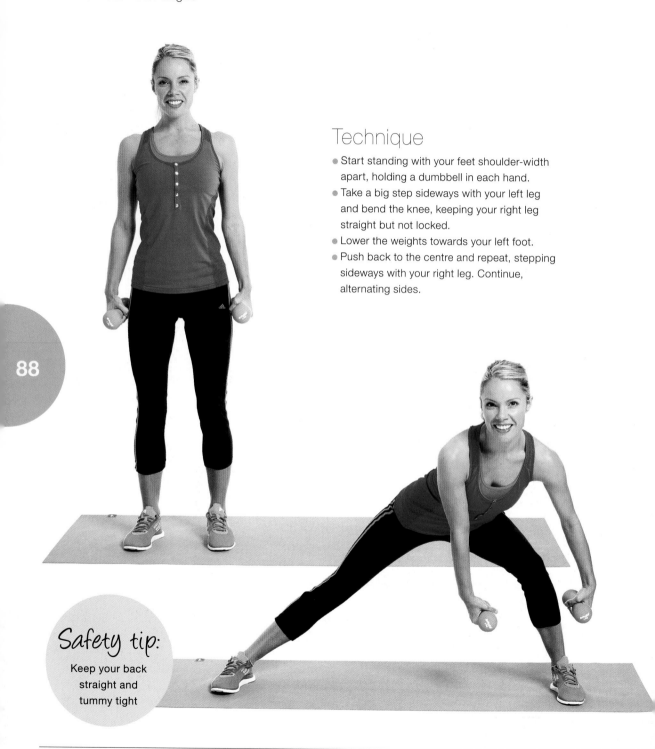

Technique

- Start standing with your feet shoulder-width apart, holding a dumbbell in each hand.
- Take a big step sideways with your left leg and bend the knee, keeping your right leg straight but not locked.
- Lower the weights towards your left foot.
- Push back to the centre and repeat, stepping sideways with your right leg. Continue, alternating sides.

88

Safety tip:
Keep your back straight and tummy tight

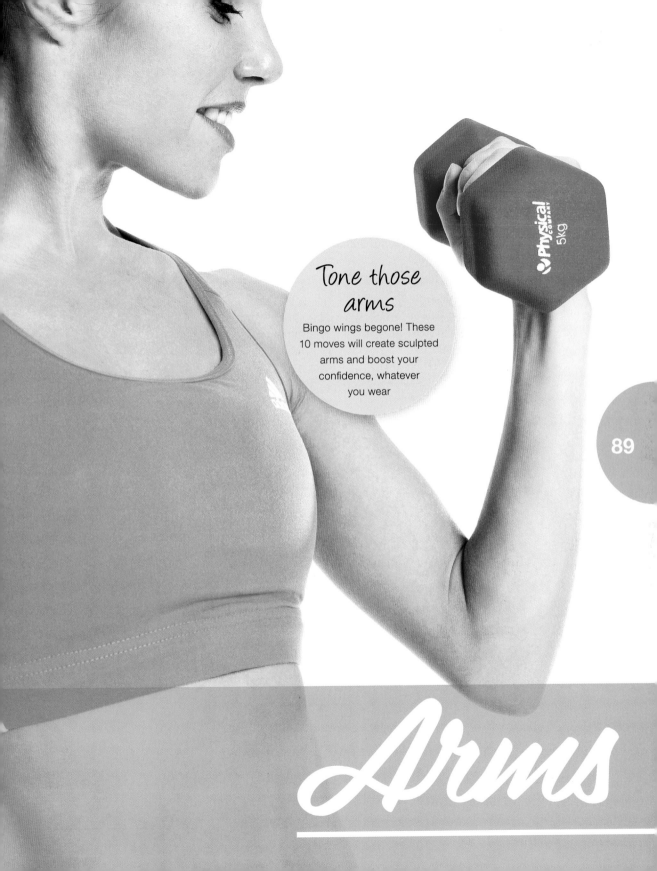

Tone those arms

Bingo wings begone! These 10 moves will create sculpted arms and boost your confidence, whatever you wear

5kg

89

Arms

Areas trained: Arms, core

Technique

- Come to the top of a press-up: resting on your hands and toes, hands directly beneath the shoulders.
- Draw the stomach towards the spine and press down through the hands to keep the arms straight. Be careful not to sag the lower back – if this begins to happen, drop the knees to the floor. Hold this pose for a count of five.
- Next, lower slowly down towards the ground, hugging the elbows in towards the rib cage, until your elbows and shoulders form a straight line just above the floor.
- Slowly return to the top of the press-up, then repeat. Advanced finish with 8 quick pulses towards the floor.
- To make the exercise easier, rest your knees on the floor.

Safety tip:

Keep your stomach muscles tight and don't allow your hips to sag

90

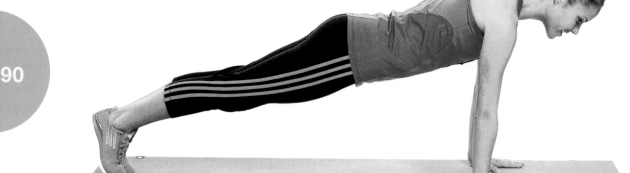

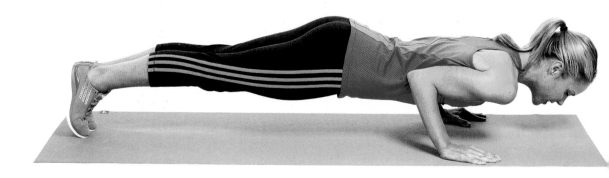

Area trained: Rear of upper arms

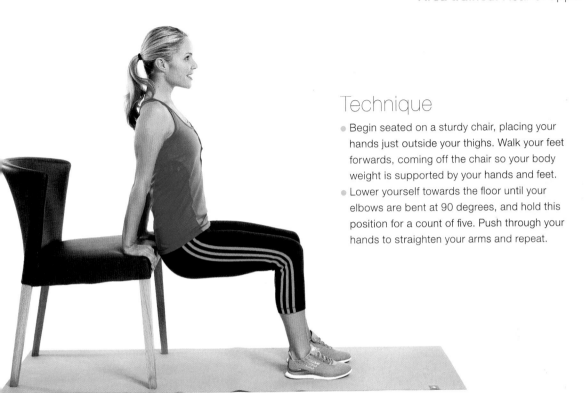

Technique

- Begin seated on a sturdy chair, placing your hands just outside your thighs. Walk your feet forwards, coming off the chair so your body weight is supported by your hands and feet.
- Lower yourself towards the floor until your elbows are bent at 90 degrees, and hold this position for a count of five. Push through your hands to straighten your arms and repeat.

Safety tip:

Keep your face forwards and your chest lifted at all times

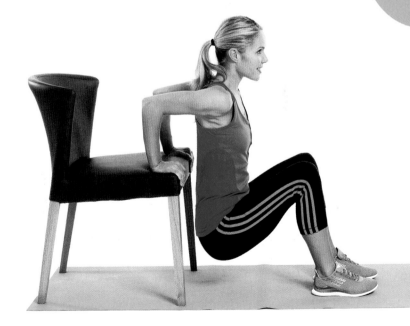

Area trained: Rear of upper arms

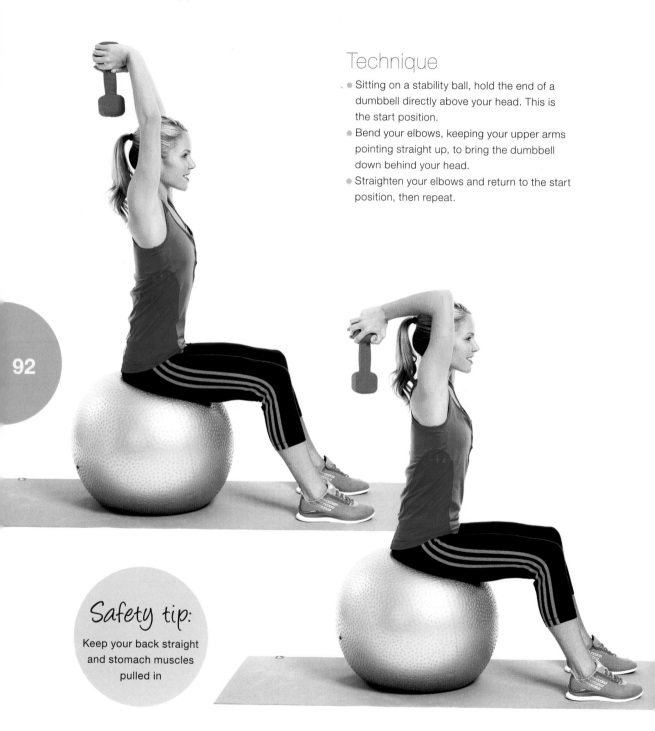

Technique

- Sitting on a stability ball, hold the end of a dumbbell directly above your head. This is the start position.
- Bend your elbows, keeping your upper arms pointing straight up, to bring the dumbbell down behind your head.
- Straighten your elbows and return to the start position, then repeat.

92

Safety tip:
Keep your back straight and stomach muscles pulled in

Areas trained: Chest, shoulders, rear of upper arms

Technique

- Begin in either a full push-up (resting on your toes) or modified push-up (resting on your knees with feet crossed, pictured) position, body in a straight line, hands under your shoulders.
- Lower your chest towards the floor, keeping your elbows close to your body, then push up, straightening your arms. Repeat for duration.

Safety tip:

Keep your back straight and stomach muscles pulled in tight

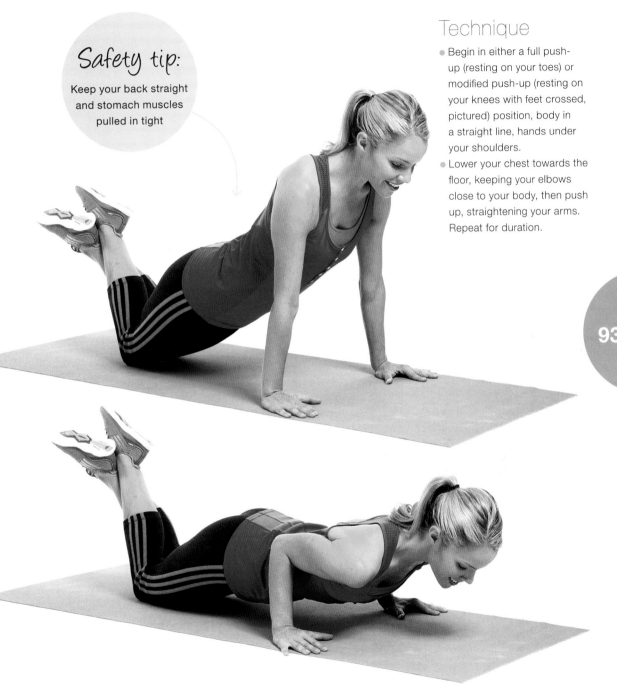

93

Areas trained: Chest, shoulders

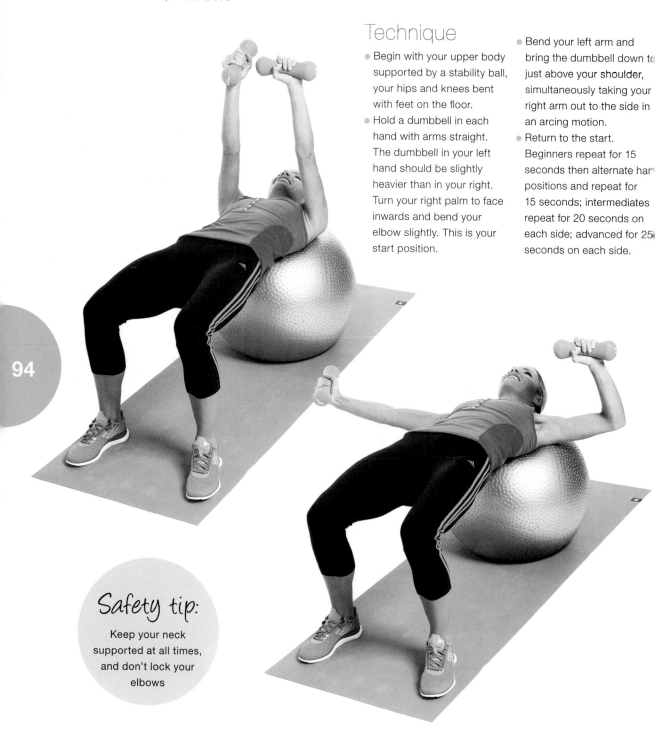

Technique

- Begin with your upper body supported by a stability ball, your hips and knees bent with feet on the floor.
- Hold a dumbbell in each hand with arms straight. The dumbbell in your left hand should be slightly heavier than in your right. Turn your right palm to face inwards and bend your elbow slightly. This is your start position.

- Bend your left arm and bring the dumbbell down to just above your shoulder, simultaneously taking your right arm out to the side in an arcing motion.
- Return to the start. Beginners repeat for 15 seconds then alternate han positions and repeat for 15 seconds; intermediates repeat for 20 seconds on each side; advanced for 25 seconds on each side.

Safety tip:
Keep your neck supported at all times, and don't lock your elbows

94

Areas trained: Chest, shoulders, rear of upper arms, core

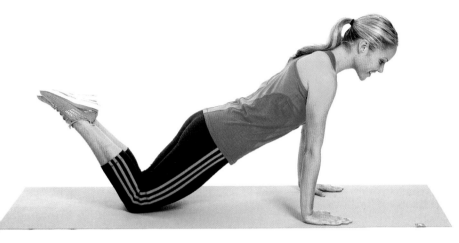

Technique

- Begin in a modified (or full) press-up position with hands directly under shoulders.
- Slowly lower your chest to the floor, keeping your elbows close to your sides.
- Straighten your arms and return to the start.
- Lift and extend your left arm and right leg so they are in line with your torso, hold for a count of one, then lower to the floor.
- Continue, alternating sides. after each press-up.

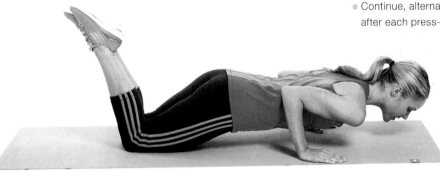

95

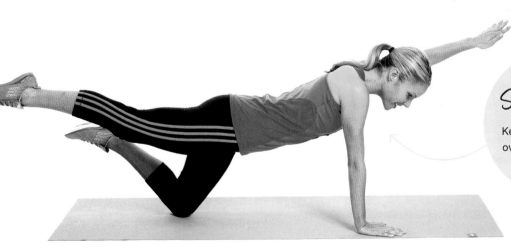

Safety tip:

Keep your shoulders over hands and your back straight

arms front and side raise

Technique

- Stand holding a dumbbell in your left hand by your side and one in your right resting on the front of your thigh, palms facing in.
- Simultaneously take your left arm out to the side and right out to the front, until your hands are level with your shoulders, keeping your elbows straight but not locked.

- Lower both arms slowly back to the start position.
- Beginners repeat for 15 seconds then alternate hand positions and repeat for a further 15 seconds; intermediates repeat for 20 seconds on each side; advanced for 25 seconds on each side.

96

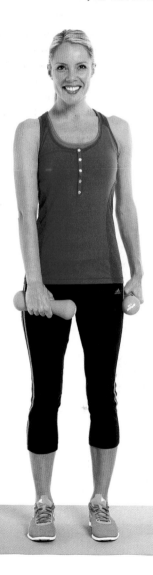

Safety tip:
Keep your back straight at all times

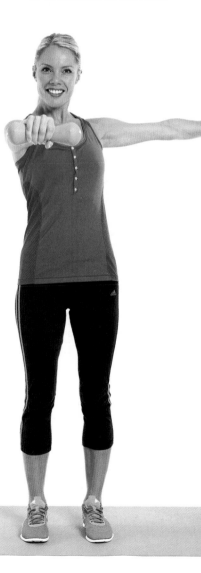

Area trained: Shoulders

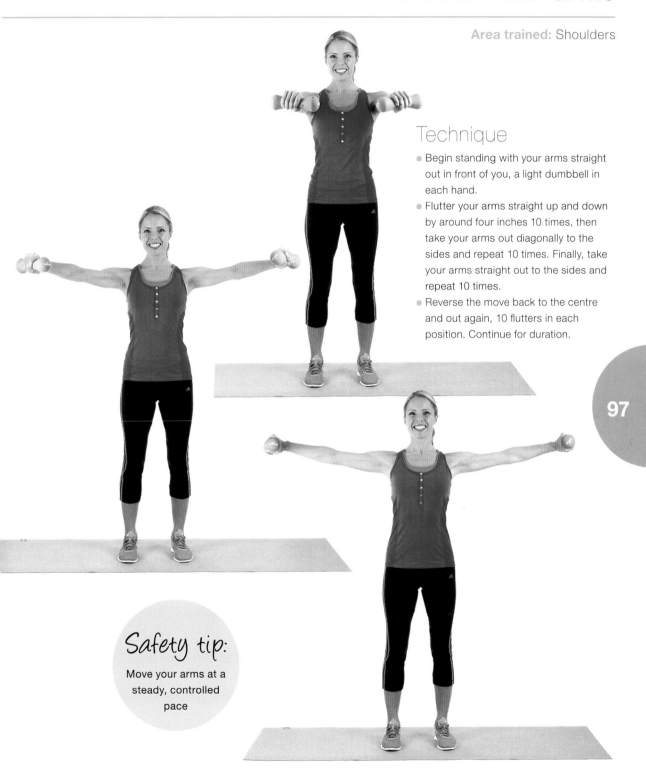

Technique

- Begin standing with your arms straight out in front of you, a light dumbbell in each hand.
- Flutter your arms straight up and down by around four inches 10 times, then take your arms out diagonally to the sides and repeat 10 times. Finally, take your arms straight out to the sides and repeat 10 times.
- Reverse the move back to the centre and out again, 10 flutters in each position. Continue for duration.

97

Safety tip:
Move your arms at a steady, controlled pace

arms row

Area trained: Upper back

Technique

- Begin standing with legs hip-width apart, holding a dumbbell in each hand.
- Bend your knees and hinge forward from the hips, so your back is parallel to the ground. Let your arms hang down in line with your shoulders with palms facing inwards. This is your start position.
- Bend your elbows so they are level with your shoulders. Slowly lower back to the start, and repeat.

98

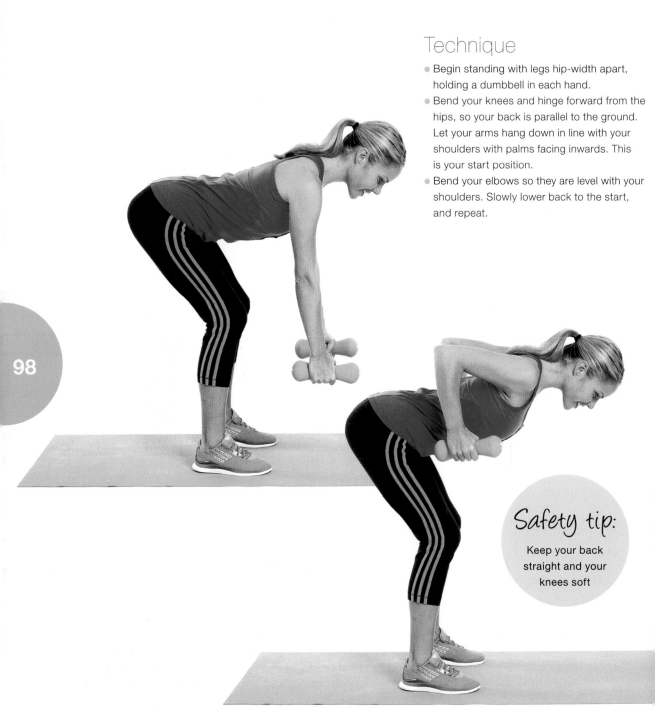

Safety tip:

Keep your back straight and your knees soft

Area trained: Front of upper arms

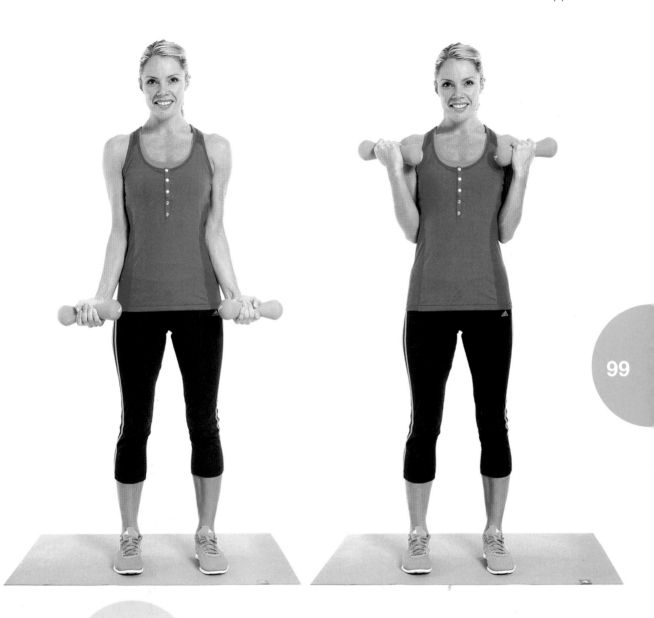

99

Safety tip:

Perform the move slowly, without momentum

Technique

- Stand with feet hip-width apart, holding dumbbells by your sides with your arms straight but not locked and palms facing away from you.

- Keeping your upper arms still and elbows by your sides, bend your elbows and bring the dumbbells towards your shoulders.
- Return slowly to the start position and repeat.

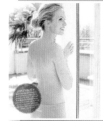

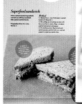
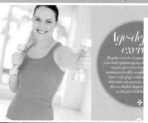
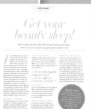
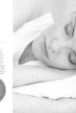

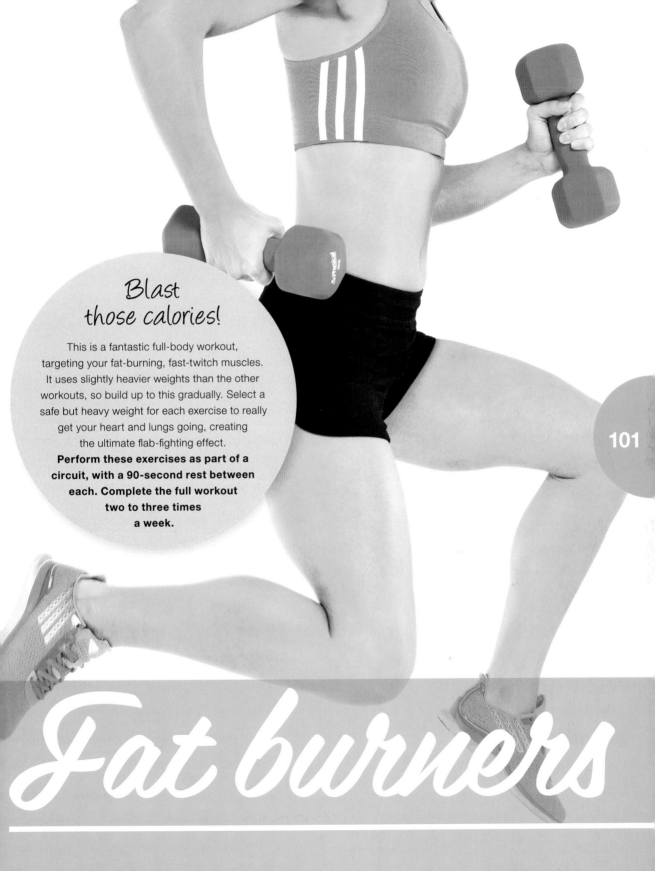

Blast those calories!

This is a fantastic full-body workout, targeting your fat-burning, fast-twitch muscles. It uses slightly heavier weights than the other workouts, so build up to this gradually. Select a safe but heavy weight for each exercise to really get your heart and lungs going, creating the ultimate flab-fighting effect. **Perform these exercises as part of a circuit, with a 90-second rest between each. Complete the full workout two to three times a week.**

Fat burners

fat burners squat press

Areas trained: Shoulders, bottom
Guidelines: Beginner 3 x 10 reps **Intermediate** 4 x 10 reps **Advanced** 5 x 10 reps

Technique

- Stand with feet shoulder-width apart, holding 6kg dumbbells either side of your face.
- Squat down as low as you can, then push up to standing, pressing the dumbbells up towards the ceiling.
- Lower the dumbbells back to the start and repeat.

Safety tip:

Avoid tipping your weight forward and overloading the knees; make sure your feet stay flat

102

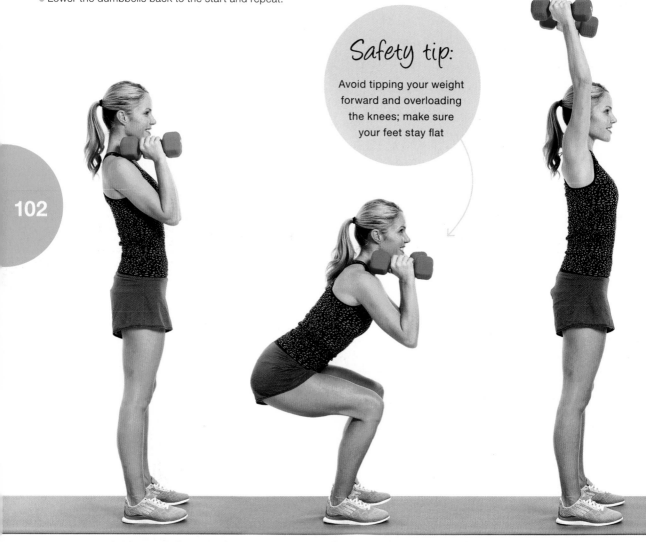

Area trained: Lower stomach

Guidelines: Beginner 3 x 10 reps **Intermediate** 4 x 10 reps **Advanced** 5 x 10 reps

Technique

- Start by resting your forearms on a stability ball, with your legs extended and your ankles, hips and shoulders in a straight line. Keep your body flat and stomach muscles tight. This is the start position.
- While keeping your body still, nudge the ball forward using your arms, before slowly returning it back to the start position.

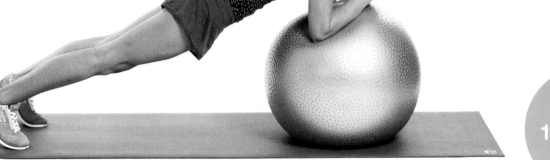

103

Safety tip:

Keep your back straight at all times

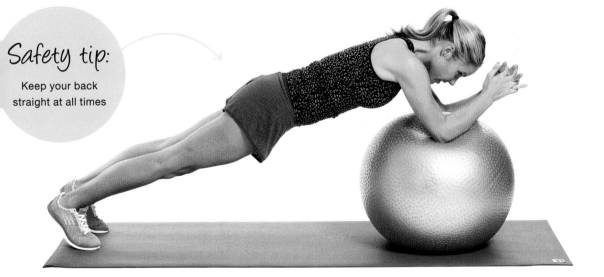

fat burners dumbbell lunge jump

Areas trained: Thighs, bottom
Guidelines: Beginner 3 x 10 reps **Intermediate** 4 x 10 reps **Advanced** 5 x 10 reps

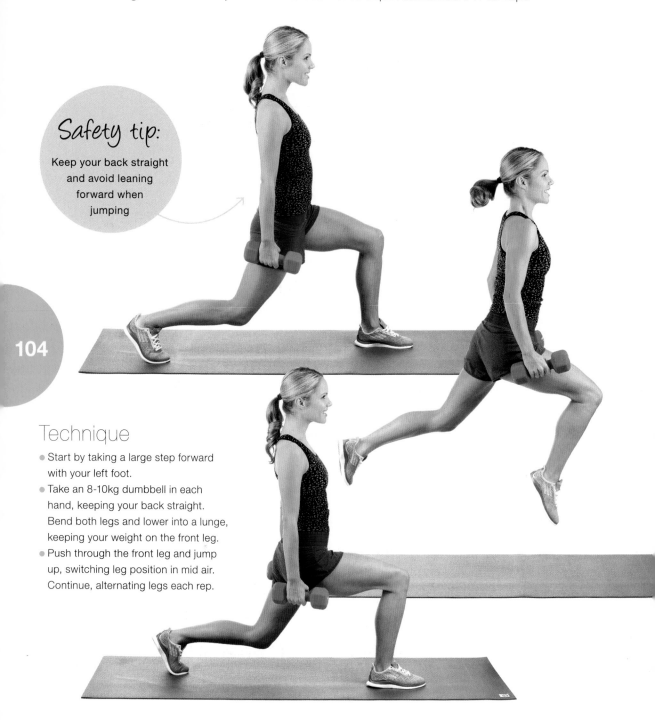

Safety tip:

Keep your back straight and avoid leaning forward when jumping

104

Technique

- Start by taking a large step forward with your left foot.
- Take an 8-10kg dumbbell in each hand, keeping your back straight. Bend both legs and lower into a lunge, keeping your weight on the front leg.
- Push through the front leg and jump up, switching leg position in mid air. Continue, alternating legs each rep.

Areas trained: Chest, rear of upper arms
Guidelines: Beginner 3 x 10 reps **Intermediate** 4 x 10 reps **Advanced** 5 x 10 reps

Technique

- Come into a plank position, resting on your toes with your hands below your shoulders.
- Lower your chest to the floor, keeping your body stiff. Slowly lift up and repeat.

Safety tip:

Keep your body in a straight line from shoulders to toes

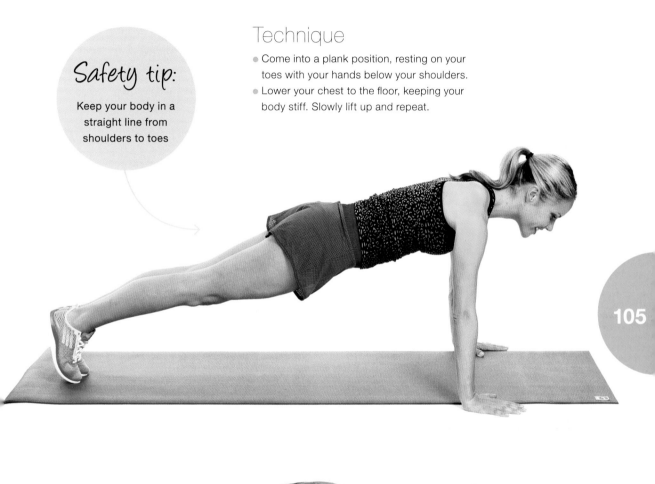

105

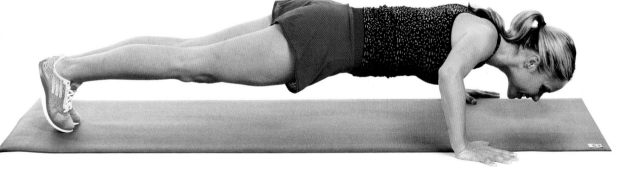

fat burners overhead oblique twists

Area trained: Side muscles
Guidelines: Beginner 3 x 10 reps each side **Intermediate** 4 x 10 reps each side
Advanced 5 x 10 reps each side

Technique

- Start by lying on your left side on a stability ball, with your left leg straight and your right foot tucked behind the left. Bring your hands to your ears, keeping the elbows wide.
- Keeping your body side-on, crunch upwards. Slowly lower back down and repeat.

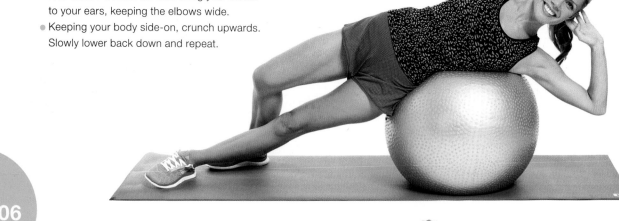

Safety tip:

Use your side muscles to lift you, don't pull on your head

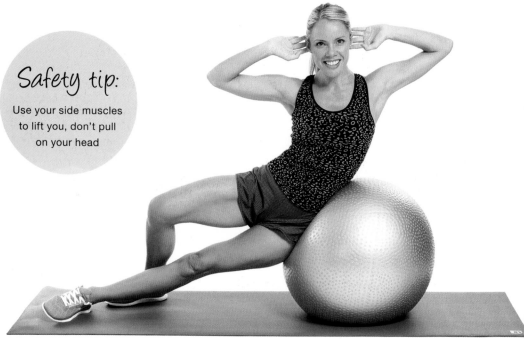

Areas trained: Back of thighs, bottom

Guidelines: Beginner 3 x 10 reps **Intermediate** 4 x 10 reps **Advanced** 5 x 10 reps

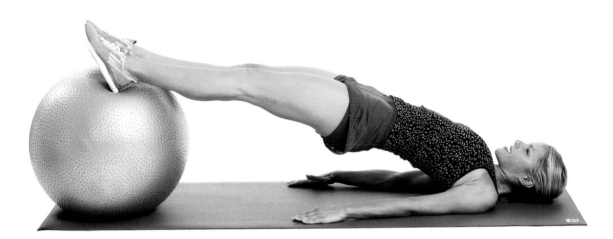

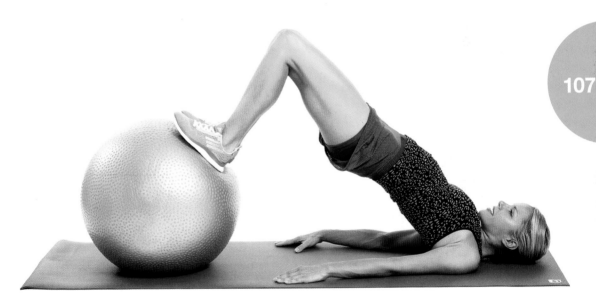

107

Technique

- Start lying on your back, feet resting on a stability ball.
- Raise your hips as high as you can towards the ceiling, this is your start position.
- Bend the knees and curl the ball towards you.
- Slowly return to the start position and repeat.

Safety tip:

Keep your stomach muscles tight at all times

fat burners stability ball knee tuck

Area trained: Stomach
Guidelines: Beginner 3 x 10 reps **Intermediate** 4 x 10 reps **Advanced** 5 x 10 reps

Safety tip:

Keep your stomach muscles tight throughout

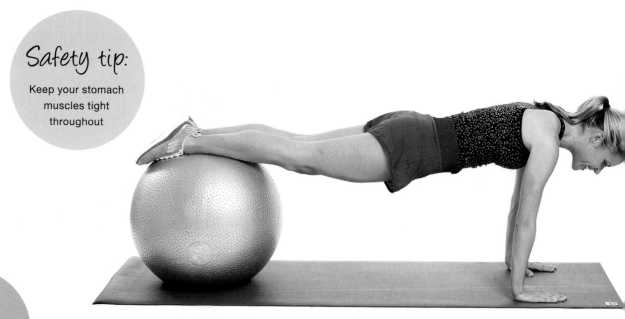

Technique

- Start with your hands on the floor, body lifted so that your shoulders are directly over your hands, feet resting on top of a stability ball.
- Keeping your upper body still and stomach muscles tight, pull the knees in towards the chest then pause for a count of one.
- Use your stomach muscles to slowly return to the start position, and repeat.

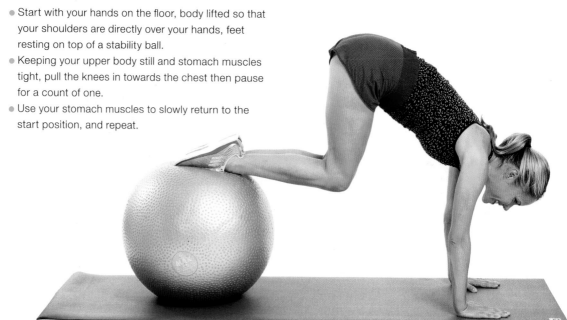

Areas trained: Upper and mid back, back of upper arms, core
Guidelines: Beginner 2 x 5 reps **Intermediate** 3 x 5 reps **Advanced** 4 x 5 reps

echnique

Come into a plank position with a 6-8kg dumbbell in each hand, palms facing each other directly under your shoulders, body resting on your toes.
Lower your chest to the floor, keeping the elbows close to the body.
Slowly lift up, keeping the body stiff. Pull one weight towards your armpit, supporting your body weight with the other arm.
Lower the weight and repeat the lift with the other arm. This counts as one rep. Repeat.

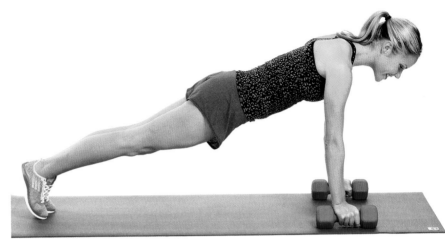

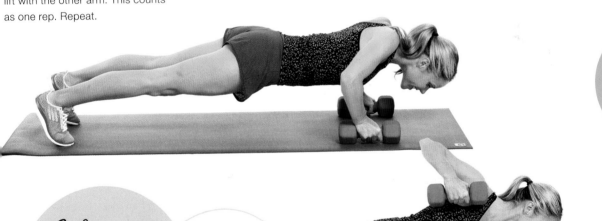

109

Safety tip:

Keep your body in a straight line from shoulders to toes. Come onto the knees if you can't maintain this form on the toes.

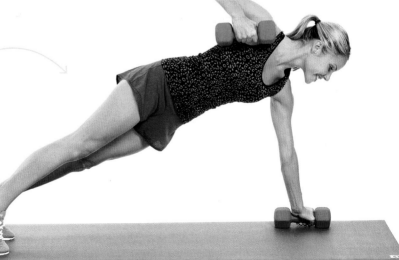

fat burners dumbbell jump squat

Areas trained: Thighs, bottom, calves, core
Guidelines: Beginner 3 x 10 reps **Intermediate** 4 x 10 reps **Advanced** 5 x 10 reps

Technique

- Stand with feet hip-width apart, holding 6-8kg dumbbells in each hand.
- Keeping your back straight and facing forwards, jump up as high as you can with an extended body.
- Land softly, then immediately squat as low as you can. Return to the start and repeat.

Safety tip:

Keep your back straight and stomach muscles pulled in tight

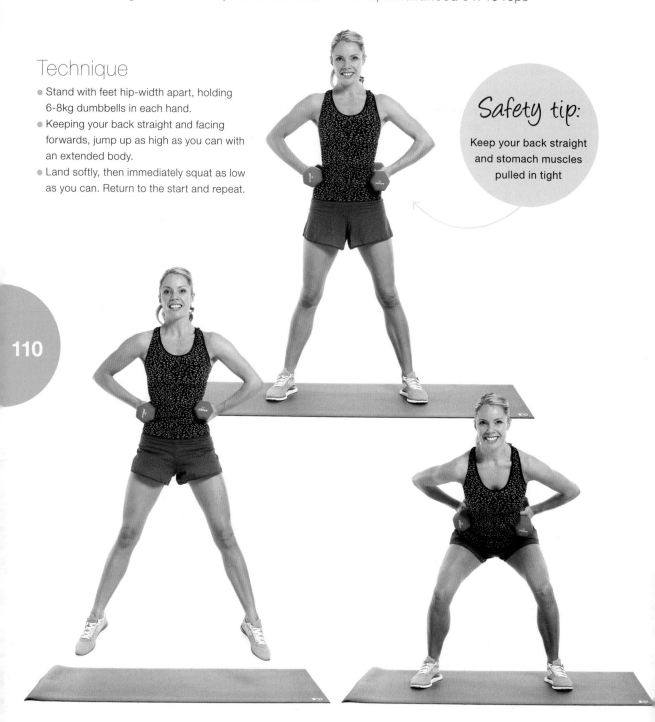

110

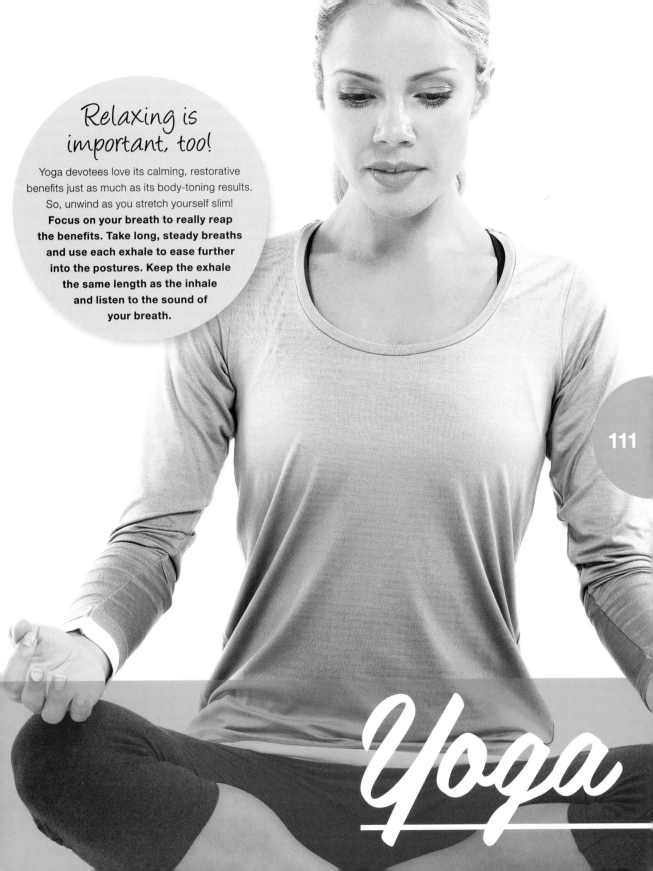

Relaxing is important, too!

Yoga devotees love its calming, restorative benefits just as much as its body-toning results. So, unwind as you stretch yourself slim! **Focus on your breath to really reap the benefits. Take long, steady breaths and use each exhale to ease further into the postures. Keep the exhale the same length as the inhale and listen to the sound of your breath.**

Yoga

yoga warrior I

Areas trained: Legs, hips, back, arms
Guidelines: Beginner 3 breaths each side **Intermediate** 5 breaths each side
Advanced 10 breaths each side

Technique

- Stand with your legs wide apart, hands by your hips. Turn your left foot out to point lengthways along the mat and pivot the right foot in slightly, to about 40 degrees. Line up your left foot with the right heel.
- Exhale, and bend the left knee to 90 degrees, in line with the left foot. Keep the right leg straight.
- Inhale, and reach the arms up to your ears, bringing your hands together in prayer position. Keep your hips square to the front and hold for the allotted breaths. Repeat on the other side.

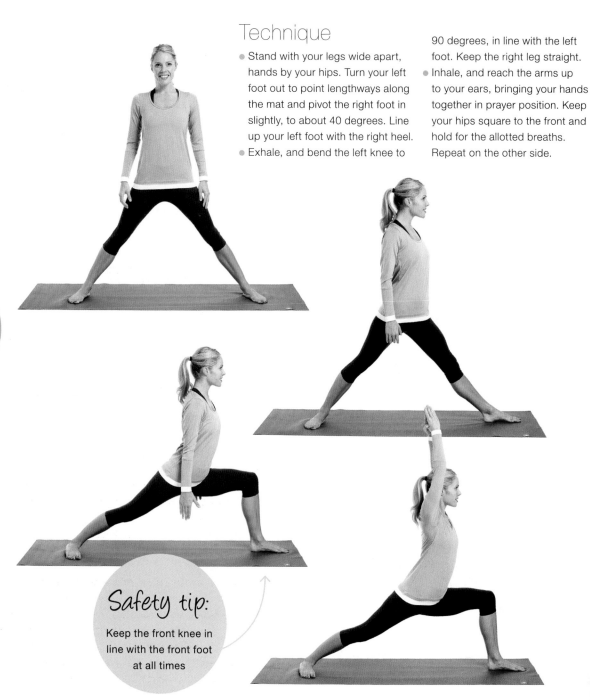

Safety tip:

Keep the front knee in line with the front foot at all times

warrior II **yoga**

Areas trained: Legs, hips, back, arms
Guidelines: Beginner 3 breaths each side **Intermediate** 5 breaths each side
Advanced 10 breaths each side

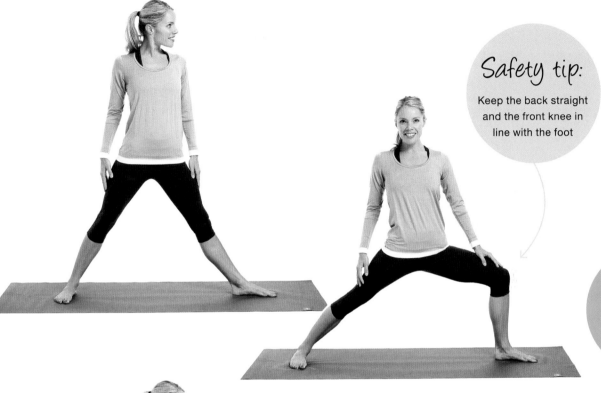

Safety tip:

Keep the back straight
and the front knee in
line with the foot

113

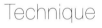

Technique

- Stand with your legs wide apart, hands by your hips. Turn your left foot out to point lengthways along the mat and pivot the right foot in slightly, to about 40 degrees. Line up your left foot with the right heel.
- Exhale, and bend the left knee to 90 degrees, keeping it in line with the left foot. Keep the right leg straight.
- Inhale, and reach the arms wide to the sides, turning your head to look past your left hand.
- Instead of letting your upper body turn towards the left, keep the hips in line with your front and back foot.
- Keep the spine straight and press the left knee to the left to keep the alignment. Lengthen the tailbone down, and hold.

yoga triangle

Areas trained: Legs, hips, back, arms
Guidelines: All levels Hold for five breaths each side

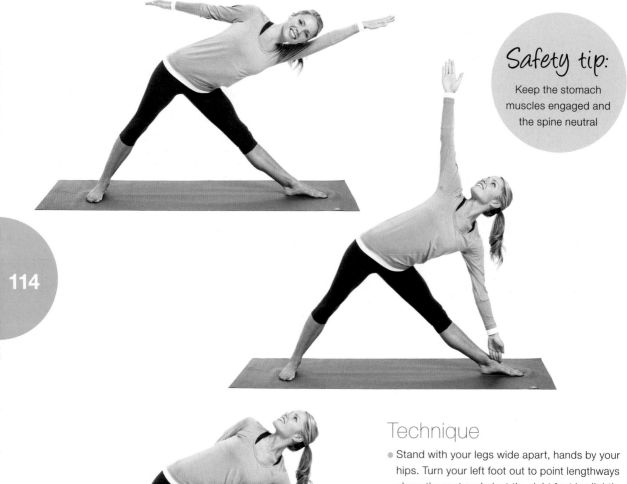

Safety tip:
Keep the stomach
muscles engaged and
the spine neutral

Technique

- Stand with your legs wide apart, hands by your hips. Turn your left foot out to point lengthways along the mat and pivot the right foot in slightly, to about 40 degrees. Line up your left foot with the right heel.
- Inhale and stretch your left arm up by the ear. Exhale and reach the left arm as far down your left leg as you can.
- Hold here, or to deepen the twist, bring your right hand behind you to your left hip. Repeat on the other side.

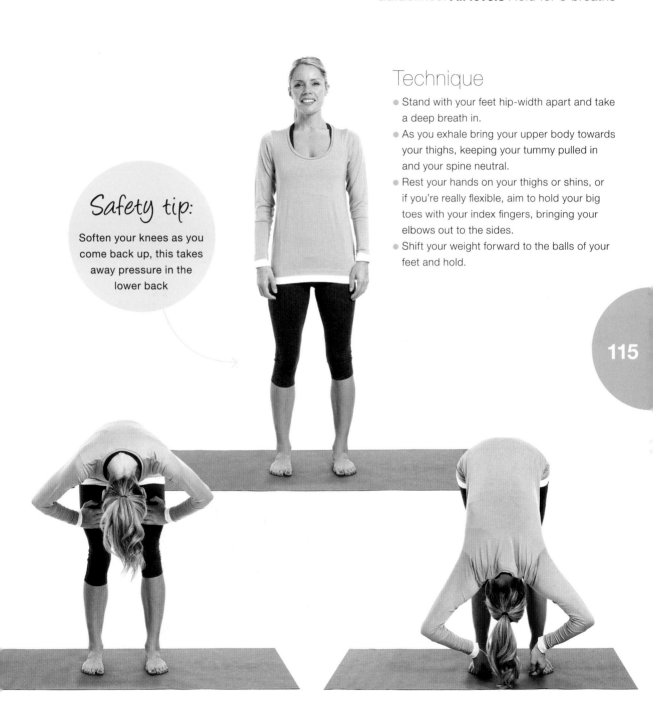

Areas trained: Legs, hips, back
Guidelines: All levels Hold for 5 breaths

Technique

- Stand with your feet hip-width apart and take a deep breath in.
- As you exhale bring your upper body towards your thighs, keeping your tummy pulled in and your spine neutral.
- Rest your hands on your thighs or shins, or if you're really flexible, aim to hold your big toes with your index fingers, bringing your elbows out to the sides.
- Shift your weight forward to the balls of your feet and hold.

Safety tip:

Soften your knees as you come back up, this takes away pressure in the lower back

115

yoga tree

Areas trained: Core stability, balance
Guidelines: Beginner 3 breaths each side **Intermediate** 5 breaths each side
Advanced 10 breaths each side

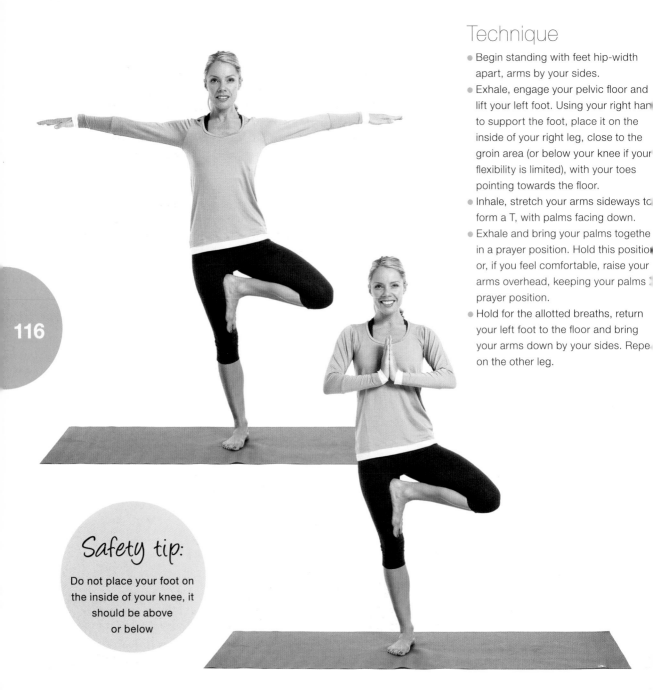

Technique

- Begin standing with feet hip-width apart, arms by your sides.
- Exhale, engage your pelvic floor and lift your left foot. Using your right hand to support the foot, place it on the inside of your right leg, close to the groin area (or below your knee if your flexibility is limited), with your toes pointing towards the floor.
- Inhale, stretch your arms sideways to form a T, with palms facing down.
- Exhale and bring your palms together in a prayer position. Hold this position or, if you feel comfortable, raise your arms overhead, keeping your palms in prayer position.
- Hold for the allotted breaths, return your left foot to the floor and bring your arms down by your sides. Repeat on the other leg.

Safety tip:

Do not place your foot on the inside of your knee, it should be above or below

Areas trained: Flexibility, back

Guidelines: Beginner 3 breaths each side **Intermediate** 5 breaths each side
Advanced 10 breaths each side

Technique

- Sit on the floor with your legs in front of you. Bend your knees and place your feet on the floor. Slide your right leg underneath your left so your right foot rests by your left buttock.
- Place your left leg over your right and place your foot on the floor by your right knee, left knee pointing towards the sky.
- Exhale and twist your body towards the left, bringing your left hand slightly behind you and your right arm to the outside of your left thigh near your knee.
- Lengthen through the torso, pressing the left foot into the ground. As you breathe in and out continue to lengthen through the spine. Hold for the required time and exhale as you release. Repeat the movement on the other side, changing legs and twisting towards the right.

117

Safety tip:

Do not pull on the knee

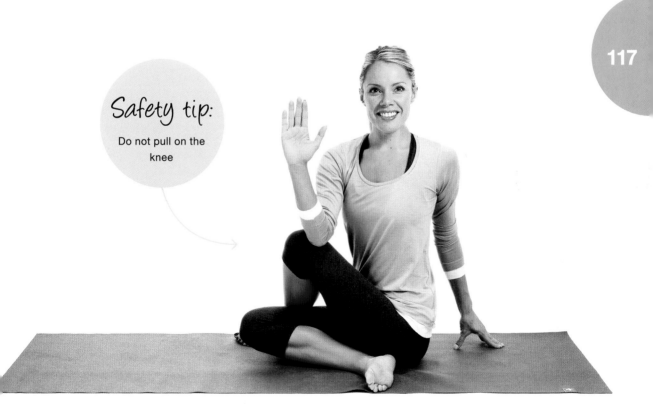

yoga cobra

Areas trained: Lower back, flexibility
Guidelines: Beginner 3 breaths **Intermediate** 5 breaths **Advanced** 10 breaths

Technique

- Lie on your front with toes pointed away, tops of feet in contact with the floor.
- Place your hands on the floor with your fingertips in line with your shoulders, elbows tucked in.
- Press the tops of the feet, thighs and pubic bone firmly into the floor.
- Lift your chest off the floor, using your back muscles rather than pressing through your hands. Stop when your elbows point straight back, and hold.

Safety tip:
Keep your feet together
and your neck relaxed
and in line with
your spine

118

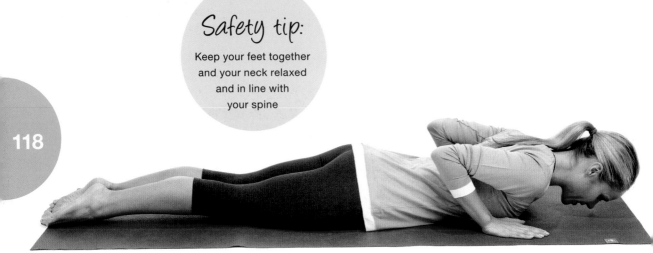

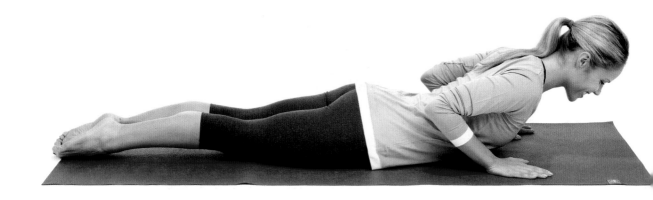

Areas trained: Shoulders, neck, hip flexors, flexibility
Repeat: Beginner 5 breaths **Intermediate** 5 breaths x 2 **Advanced** 5 breaths x 3

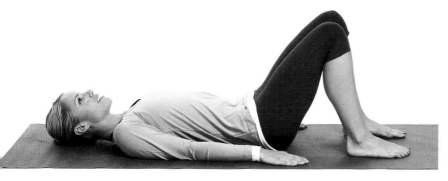

Technique

- Lie flat on your back, legs hip-width apart, with your arms by your side, palms down. Bend your knees, and bring your feet on the floor as close to you bum as possible.
- Lift your hips, pressing through your feet, and clasp your hands together below your pelvis.
- Take deep breaths into your ribs rather than your stomach.

Safety tip:

Keep your head straight and neck relaxed

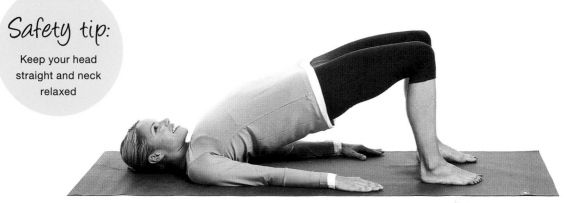

119

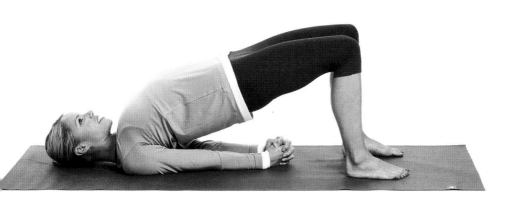

yoga savasana

Area trained: Whole-body relaxation
Guidelines: All levels 5-10 minutes

Technique

- Lie on your back, feet hip-width apart and relaxed outwards. Place your arms 45 degrees away from your body, palms facing up.
- Close your eyes and relax.

120

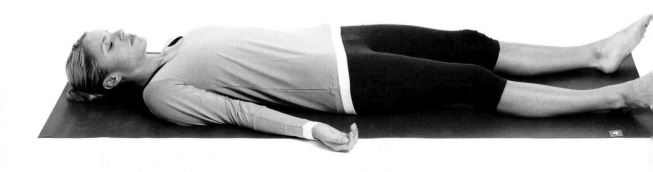

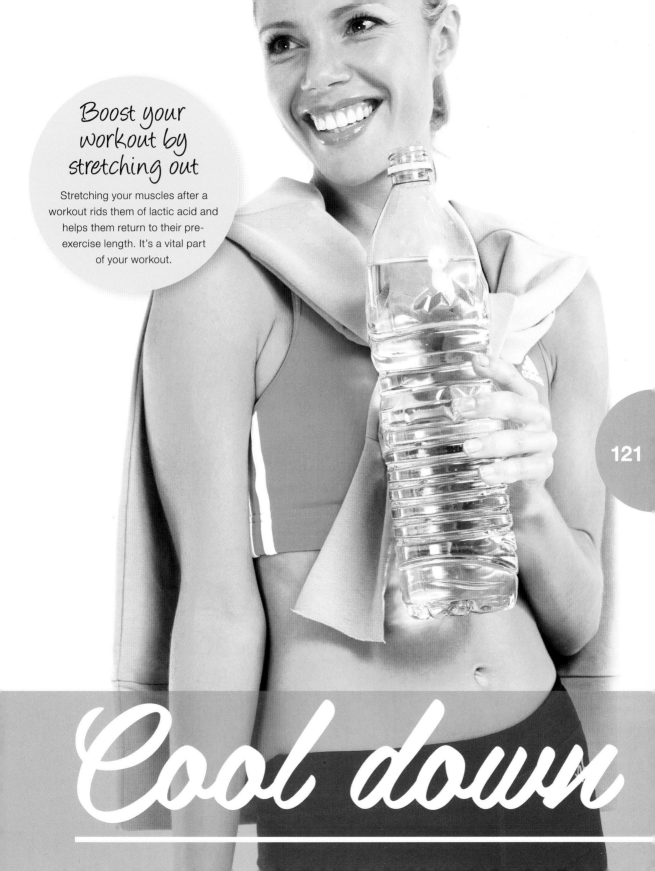

Boost your workout by stretching out

Stretching your muscles after a workout rids them of lactic acid and helps them return to their pre-exercise length. It's a vital part of your workout.

121

Cool down

cool down butterfly stretch

Area stretched: Inner thighs
Guidelines: All levels hold for 20-30 seconds

Technique

- Sit on the floor with legs bent and soles of the feet together, as close to the body as comfortable.
- Hold the ankles with your hands and use your forearms to push down on the inner thighs, bringing the knees towards the floor.

Safety tip:

Keep the core tight and back straight

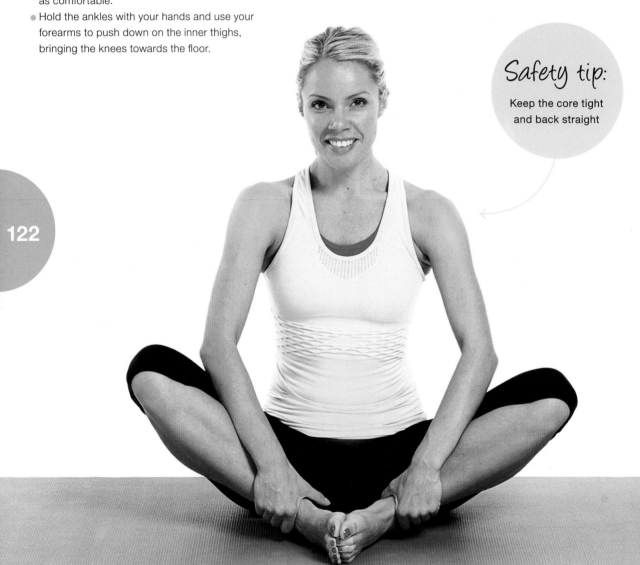

Area stretched: Bottom
Guidelines: All levels hold for 10-15 seconds

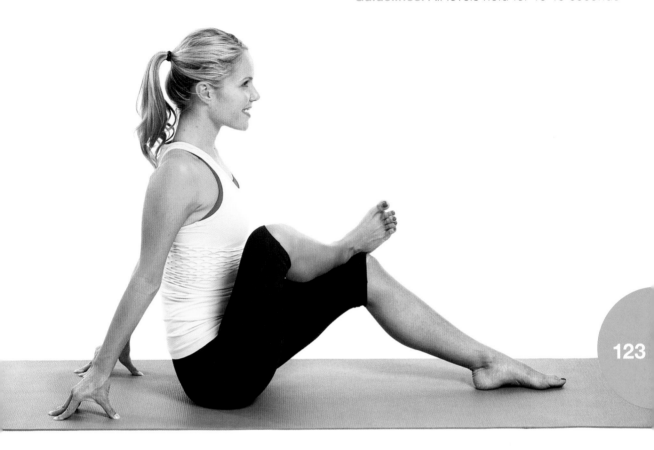

123

Technique

- Sit on the floor leaning back slightly, with knees at a 90-degree angle and feet flat on the floor. Place your hands behind you to support your weight.
- Rest your right ankle across the top of your left thigh so that your right knee is pointing outwards and the lower leg is parallel to the floor.
- Apply pressure by bringing your body closer to your leg. Hold, then repeat on the other side.

Safety tip:

Keep your chest lifted and don't arch your back

Area stretched: Front of thighs
Guidelines: All levels hold for 10-15 seconds

Technique

- Lie face down on the floor, with forehead resting on your left forearm for comfort.
- Bending your leg, bring your right foot to your right buttock and hold the foot with your right hand for support. Hold, then repeat on the other leg.

124

Safety tip:

Don't pull too hard on the bent leg

Area stretched: Back of thighs
Guidelines: All levels hold for 20-30 seconds

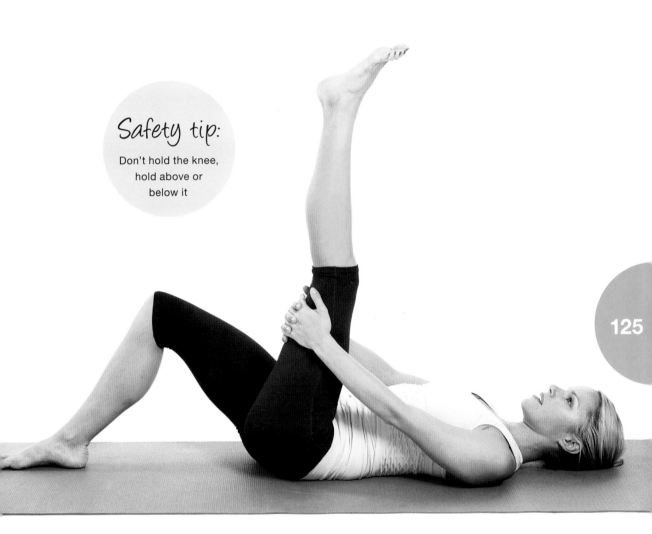

Safety tip:

Don't hold the knee,
hold above or
below it

125

Technique

- Lie on your back and bend the right leg to a right angle so the foot is flat on the floor.
- Keeping your left leg straight, elevate it and take hold of the back of the thigh or calf with both hands.
- Pull gently towards the body, keeping the leg straight. Hold, then repeat on the other leg.

cool down lying abdominal stretch

Area stretched: Stomach
Guidelines: All levels hold for 10-15 seconds

Technique

- Lie face down on the floor and place your hands on either side of your body.
- Push your torso upwards, and rest on your forearms, keeping the hips on the floor.

Safety tip:

Keep your chest lifted and your shoulders square

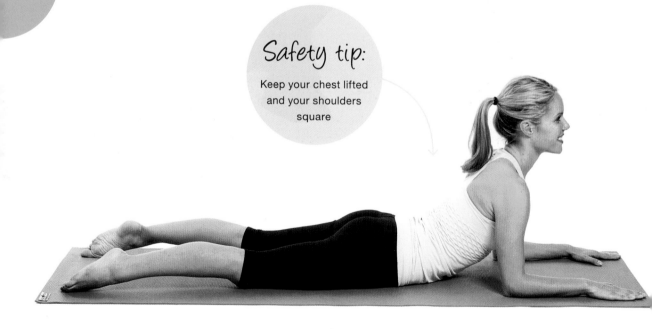

Area stretched: Lower back
Guidelines: All levels hold for 20-30 seconds

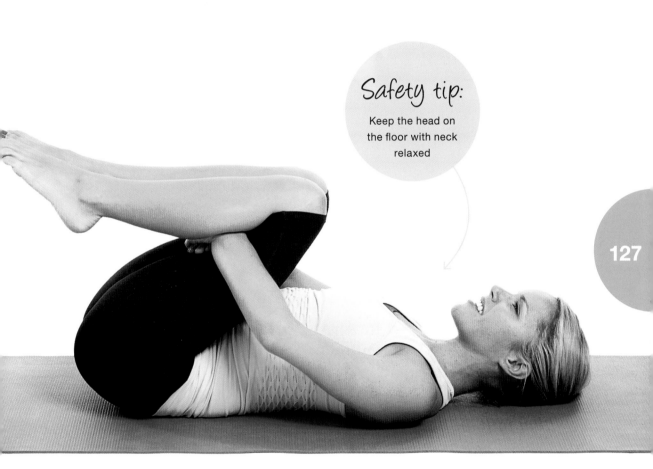

Safety tip:

Keep the head on
the floor with neck
relaxed

127

Technique

- Lying with your back on the floor, bring your knees to your chest.
- Place hands around the backs of your thighs to gently pull your knees further towards you.

cool down seated chest stretch

Areas stretched: Chest, front of shoulders
Guidelines: All levels hold for 20-30 seconds

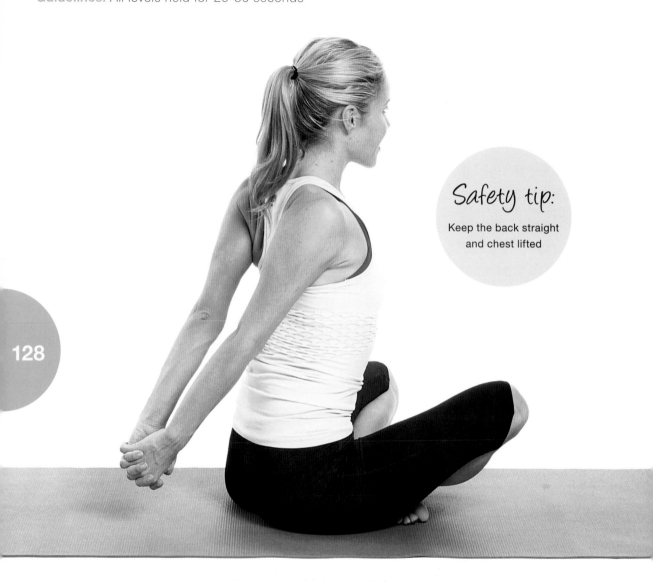

Safety tip:
Keep the back straight
and chest lifted

128

Technique

- Sit down cross-legged and place your hands on the small of your lower back.
- Clasp your hands and bring them straight out behind you.

Area stretched: Back
Guidelines: All levels hold for 10-15 seconds

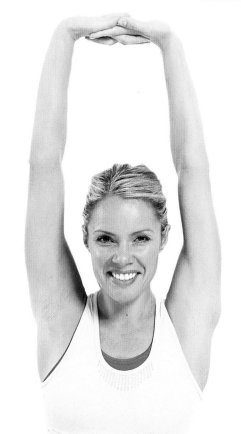

Technique

- Sit down and stretch your arms above your head, with one hand clasping the other, palms facing away from you.
- Reach upwards.

129

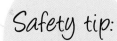

Safety tip:

Keep your back straight

cool down seated deltoid stretch

Areas stretched: Shoulders, rear of upper arms
Guidelines: All levels hold for 10-15 seconds

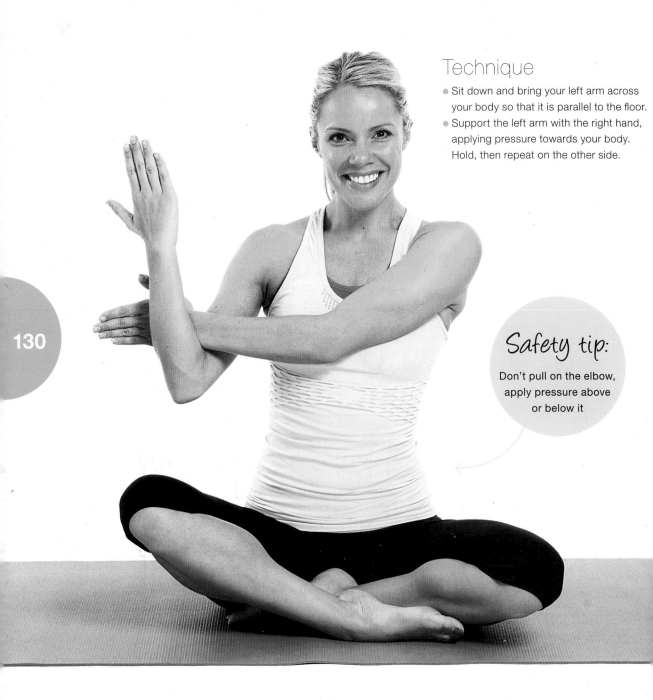

Technique

- Sit down and bring your left arm across your body so that it is parallel to the floor.
- Support the left arm with the right hand, applying pressure towards your body. Hold, then repeat on the other side.

Safety tip:
Don't pull on the elbow, apply pressure above or below it

130